Swara Yoga

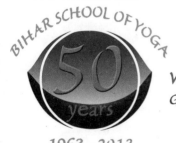

WORLD YOGA CONVENTION 2013
GANGA DARSHAN, MUNGER, BIHAR, INDIA
23rd–27th October 2013

1963–2013
GOLDEN JUBILEE

Swara Yoga
The Tantric Science of Brain Breathing

Including the original Sanskrit text of the
Shiva Swarodaya with English translation

Swami Muktibodhananda

Under the Guidance of
Swami Satyananda Saraswati

Yoga Publications Trust, Munger, Bihar, India

Published by Bihar School of Yoga
    First edition 1984
    Reprinted 1999

Published by Yoga Publications Trust
    Reprinted 2004, 2005, 2008, 2009, 2014

ISBN: 978-81-85787-36-7

Publisher and distributor: Yoga Publications Trust, Ganga Darshan, Munger, Bihar, India.

Website: www.biharyoga.net
         www.rikhiapeeth.net

Printed at Thomson Press (India) Limited, New Delhi, 110001

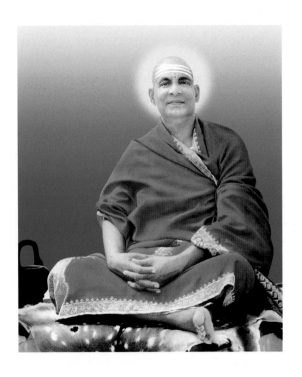

Dedication

In humility we offer this dedication to
Swami Sivananda Saraswati, who initiated
Swami Satyananda Saraswati into the secrets of yoga.

Contents

Shiva Swarodaya

Swara Yoga in Theory

Swami Satyananda Saraswati on Swara Yoga

For thousands of years mankind has been attempting to penetrate the realm of inner experience. Every thinking person has tried his level best to accomplish this great task. Thus there are many different ways and means to have the inner experience, and from time to time man has experimented with the various paths. Some talk about karma yoga, others about bhakti yoga, raja yoga, jnana yoga, kundalini yoga, etc. Quite a few have also ventured to develop inner experience through the use of drugs.

Many people say that only those who are perfected can have inner experience, but yoga says it is the right of everybody. Perfect or imperfect, theist or atheist, high born or low born, all can have that experience. Therefore, many systems of yoga have been devised. Out of all these systems, tantra can be distinguished separately because it is the path of total transcendence whereby you can have that experience in spite of any limitation or barrier. In the tantric tradition some aspects are widely known while others are almost forgotten. Amongst the latter is the science of swara yoga.

Swara yoga is the ancient science of pranic body rhythms which explains how the movement of prana can be controlled by manipulation of the breath. Recently modern science has taken great interest in electromagnetic fields and the behaviour of bioenergy, which is the inherent energy principle of the body. With eyciting developments accelerating in such areas as bioenergetics, psychotronics and Kirlian photography, the science of swara yoga is now in great demand.

Although swara yoga is still practised in India, it is not well known, either in the East or in the West. Perhaps this is because it was always regarded as an esoteric science which could possibly harm people if improperly practised. The tradition was preserved secretly by experienced yogis who handed it down in strict accordance with the rules of practice.

Previously, in fact, swara yoga was even more closely guarded than most of the other tantric traditions. Initiation was only given by direct transmission or by word of mouth from guru to disciple. Consequently, little was ever written down regarding the finer aspects of the theory and practice. For this reason, we find few references to the subject even in the yogic and tantric texts, and very little is available in English translation.

Swara etymologically means 'the sound of one's own breath'. *Yoga* means 'union'. Therefore, swara yoga enables the state of union to be reached by means of one's breath. Through the practice of swara yoga, one can realize the breath as being the medium of the cosmic life force. The breath has so much importance in human existence that the ancient rishis or seers evolved a complete science around it just from studying the simple process of respiration.

Swara yoga, however, should not be confused with pranayama, which involves a different aspect of the breath. Although both deal with prana, swara yoga emphasizes the analysis of the breath and the significance of different pranic rhythms, whereas pranayama involves techniques to redirect, store and control prana. Swara yoga may therefore be said to involve the practices of pranayama, but in fact it is a much more extensive and precise science.

Many of the yogic texts such as *Shiva Samhita* and *Goraksha Samhita* and various Upanishads discuss the functions of prana. However, the main source of recorded knowledge on swara yoga comes from the *Shiva Swarodaya*. *Shiva* is the supreme consciousness. *Swara* is the breath flow and *udaya*

4

means waking or rising. This text extols the significance of the different types of breath or pranic rhythms as told by Lord Shiva.

In the tantric tradition Lord Shiva, who is known as *Adinath* (the primordial guru), first expounded the knowledge of swara to his disciple, Parvati or Devi. The *Shiva Swarodaya* was the outcome of this dialogue. The very opening of the *Shiva Swarodaya* emphasizes the importance of swara yoga. Shiva implores Devi to make sure that the science is kept very secret and sacred, and remains the highest of all the *vidyas* or forms of knowledge. Lord Shiva further states that in all the seven lokas he knows no greater wisdom or treasure than the swara.

According to the swara shastras, by analysis of the breath deeper understanding of the cosmos is unfolded and the wisdom revealed within the Vedas can be realized. Through knowledge of the swara, a sadhaka can become a perfected yogi.

The physical act of breathing is said to have a very subtle influence on the level of consciousness and therefore the effects of swara yoga are also very subtle. It aims at directly awakening the highest human potential. In other systems a similar understanding of the swara of the breath is also expressed. For example, in Taoism it states that, "If one meditates upon the breath, the cosmic deities or forces can be seen operating in the physical body. By sustaining oneself purely on the breath, rather than on coarse food, one's entire being will be purified and strengthened. Then the consciousness is able to ascend to the heavens where eternal life is experienced by the body and soul."

Swara yoga not only helps those who believe in a supreme reality, but also those who do not have faith and who will also be surprised to discover many truths pertaining to this reality. Swara yoga is a path which leads to total experience and awakening of the entire being.

There are a number of things concerning swara yoga which need to be understood before the practice can be applied correctly. It involves many aspects of the breathing process. You have to know about the movement of prana in the body and its relationship with the mind. Prana manifests in different ways and has particular effects on each organ and part of the system. When you understand this, you can predict forthcoming events or cure your illnesses.

There are many techniques for controlling the swara so that during the day the left nostril remains active and prana moves in a particular direction. Or by making the prana flow through the right nostril during the night you can create another type of energy movement and stimulus, so that you can have a good sleep without tranquillizers, work the whole day without becoming fatigued, or you can digest food without taking appetisers or digestives. These are all different aspects of swara yoga.

In fact, if someone comes to you with a question which you cannot answer, you will be able to answer it correctly by studying the particular flow of the swara. Of course, you must be careful as you may make a wrong calculation if the breath is disturbed. But just as an example, if the person who is questioning approaches from the side opposite to the flowing swara, the answer has to be no, and if he approaches on the side of the active swara, the answer has to be yes.

This is only to give you an idea of the diverse field of the science; it is not the most important part of swara yoga. This aspect relates to mundane life, and ultimately it must be transcended. You must be able to realize how prana manifests in all forms and that everything in creation is due to pranic movement. For example, you may practise hatha yoga to improve your strength and vitality, but that is not the ultimate purpose, it is only a side effect. Likewise, the various techniques of swara yoga can be useful in mundane affairs; however, the actual purpose is to enable you to realize the true essence of your being and to unfold the inner experience.

1

Swara Yoga in Brief

When we use the word 'swara', we are talking about something more than the air which flows from the nostrils, we are also talking about the flow of prana, a very subtle and vital aspect of the breath. Up to now, knowledge of the swara has only been sought by a small minority of people. In fact, breathing is a process which is generally ignored, although it is the most important function of the body.

Breathing continues twenty-four hours a day, whether one is aware of it or not. The breath is man's most valuable treasure because without it he cannot exist for more than three minutes. There is a saying that man is born alone and dies alone, but this is incorrect. Man is born with his breath, and with his subtle prana, which is the essence of the breath, he departs. Breath is man's 'soul' companion. Therefore, the Upanishads refer to swara as atmaswaroopa or brahmaswaroopa, thus inferring that man is a part of Brahman or the universal consciousness. If you can realize the true reality of the breath, you can realize the *atma* or soul.

Breathing is therefore more than a simple physical action. Each breath has an underlying significance and a particular 'coded message'. For the spiritual aspirant the breath provides a vehicle by which he can reach the ultimate goal. Ordinary breathing is a mechanical function performed by the physical body, but in swara yoga breathing is a process which can be manipulated and controlled.

The alternating breath

If you ever take the time to observe the breath and the manner in which the air flows in and out of the nostrils, you will notice that most of the time respiration takes place through one nostril only. It appears that respiration occurs through both nostrils simultaneously, but this is not so. When you observe the breath, you will find that one nostril usually remains open for a certain duration of time and the breath comes and goes through that side only. Later this nostril closes and the alternate nostril opens.

What does this mean? Physiologically, it has a particular effect on the nervous system, producing a certain type of stimulus. Furthermore, it has a specific influence on the brain which requires very systematic regulation. Swara yoga is the science which reveals this previously unknown process.

Swara yoga explains how the flow of the swara changes at regular intervals; it is not at all erratic. Every hour or every hour and twenty minutes the active nostril changes. This rhythm regulates all the psychological and physiological processes. If the swara is irregular, it is a clear indication that something is not functioning properly in the body.

The three swaras

The fact that we breathe alternately is very significant in swara yoga because it allows different swaras to flow at different times. One swara flows through the left nostril, another flows through the right, and the third flows through both nostrils together. The different swaras influence us in various ways by stimulating different energy centres and aspects of the nervous system.

In fact, it is not just by chance that the swara flows sometimes through the right nostril and at other times through the left. The rhythm of the body is based on the biorhythms, the energy rhythms of the body, and it also relates to the two hemispheres of the brain.

In the human body the three swaras correspond to the three major systems, which can be termed as a trinity. Mind is one aspect, life force is another and spirit or soul is the third. Mind, life force and spirit combined constitute the human being. In swara yoga, mind is known as *chitta*, life force as *prana* and spirit as *atma*. Chitta controls the sensory nerves: the eyes, nose, tongue, ears and skin. Prana controls the five organs of action: speech, hands, feet, reproductive and urinary/excretory organs. Atma is the overall witness or controller.

When the left nostril flows, it indicates that the mental energy, chitta, is predominant, and the pranic energy is weak. When the right nostril flows, the pranic forces are stronger and the mental aspect is weak. When both nostrils operate together, it indicates that the spiritual energy, the force of the atma, is in power.

Action in relation to swara

Swara yoga enables us to understand the nature of the breath and its influence on the body because the different swaras lead to different types of action, mental, physical and spiritual. When you are meditating, praying or contemplating the truth, it is spiritual action. When you are walking, talking, urinating or eating, it is physical action. When digestion is going on and the enzymes are flowing in the body, it is physical action. But when you are worried or have many thoughts on your mind, or when you are memorizing a poem or song, or planning something, it is mental action. Whether you have compassion in your mind or you are angry with somebody, it is all mental action. These are just a few examples of the three categories of action.

All of our actions can be classified into three main categories, and each type of action is presided over by a specific flow of the swara. The left swara presides over mental actions, the right swara over physical actions, and both swaras together preside over spiritual actions. This means that if the right nostril flows when you are meditating, you will have physical difficulties. The body will be restless. If the left nostril is flowing, you may not be physically disturbed,

9

but the mind will wander. However, when both nostrils are open, the mind becomes one-pointed. Then you can easily become absorbed in the process of meditation.

Therefore, in swara yoga the first rule is correct action for the appropriate swara. For this purpose you will have to train yourself to maintain control over the swara according to the action you are performing, or you should adjust your action to suit the swara. Thus, swara yoga aims at harmonizing the mind and body by adjusting the actions with the swara.

Ida, pingala and sushumna

We have been talking about the flow of the breath, which creates a flow of energy in the body. The word for flow in yoga is *nadi*. In the nostrils three different flows of energy are created. These are known as *ida, pingala* and *sushumna*. The left nostril is connected to the ida network of nadis, the right nostril to pingala, and when both nostrils function together, the main channel or sushumna network is stimulated.

The energy flows created by the left and right swaras act something like the positive and negative currents in an electrical circuit. The left swara is the negative line, while the right is the positive. When the right nostril is flowing, it is said that pingala stimulates the body. When the left nostril is flowing, ida stimulates the mental faculties. During the time when the swara is alternating, both nostrils become active simultaneously. Then sushumna nadi is said to stimulate the atma or spiritual potential. But this usually occurs only during the period of changeover for a couple of minutes.

Sushumna nadi is the cause of spiritual actions and it is the purpose of every yogic and tantric system to activate it. Sushumna runs straight up the centre of the spine and merges with ida and pingala a little above the nasal root at ajna chakra, the point behind the eyebrow centre. It is through sushumna that the kundalini shakti, the high-

10

powered spiritual force, has to be channelled. When both nostrils are active, it is an indication that the sushumna passage is open. Therefore, equalizing the breath is important for it is associated with the opening of sushumna nadi.

When sushumna flows, the mental and physical energy patterns become even and rhythmic, the thoughts are stilled and the mind is calm. Therefore, it is also known as the shoonya swara. *Shoonya* means void. For the yogi this is the most significant type of swara because it aids in the practice of *dhyana* or meditation. The aim of swara yoga is therefore to develop the shoonya swara by reducing the activities of the alternating breath.

Breathing goes deeper than the lungs

What is the significance of the flow of each swara and why does it change? This is what swara yoga aims to answer. In the swara shastras it says that personal and detailed knowledge of one's swara can only be had from the guru. But the shastras do give us some hints. They say that swara is prana, the vital energy force. It is the medium for transmission of prana shakti throughout the whole body. Therefore, it affects more than just the gross plane of existence. It is most important in the subtle and spiritual realms.

The *Mundaka Upanishad* compares the swara to a bowstring on which the consciousness can be raised to pierce the atman or universal spirit. Breathing not only maintains the physical body, it is a direct medium for the evolution of consciousness. As far as medical science is concerned, it is connected with the purely organic function of the respiratory system. That is correct, but swara yoga offers a deeper insight than this, because man's existence does not begin and end with the physical body. Beyond the physical body exists energy; beyond energy, mind; beyond mind, consciousness; beyond consciousness, superconsciousness. Swara yoga, therefore, studies the flow of energy in order to enable us to come closer to realizing the depth and immensity of the mind, consciousness and cosmos.

11

2

Prana: Vital Energy

In swara yoga, as in all other yogas, importance is given to the theoretical as well as the practical aspects of the breath. According to the *Shiva Swarodaya*: "One has to know about prana and its variations, the nadis or energy pathways, and the different tattwas or elements of the macrocosmos. Through the application of such knowledge, the swara yogi can know all the events of the universe which are both auspicious and inauspicious. He will come to realize that the shakti of the swara, inherent prana, is functioning throughout the whole of creation, and that ultimately even the form of Lord Shiva is the swara, the breath and the prana."

Individual and cosmic prana

In most of the yogic texts the term prana is associated with life force or bioenergy. Many people even use the word prana for oxygen, confusing it with the subdivision of prana vayu which regulates the heart and lungs. But when we speak of prana in the higher sense, we are referring to the cosmic concept rather than the physical breath or the atmospheric ions. Life in itself is not a gross concept, and just because something exists does not mean it represents prana.

Prana is a Sanskrit word derived from two roots: *pra* is a prefix used to denote constancy and *na* means 'movement'.

12

Therefore, prana is a force in constant motion, like a vibration moving to and fro without any interception. We have to be very precise when we use the word prana, because it has two aspects – cosmic and individual. Cosmic prana is very subtle and can only be perceived by the infinite mind, but individual prana related to the body is grosser and more tangible. In the order of creation, prana emanates from the unmanifest reality known as *hiranyagarbha*, the golden womb or egg. On the physical level it manifests as individual existence. Swara yoga develops awareness of the manifestation and existence of prana within our own being so that we can come to realize its cosmic propensity.

The inherent energy of the breath

In yoga, breathing is considered to be a very important process because it is the most vital means of absorbing prana into the body. The shastras explain how prana gives consciousness and life to every creature which breathes. In the *Taittiriya, Brahmana* and *Maitri Upanishads* and *Shiva Swarodaya*, the breath is referred to as the vehicle of Brahman or cosmic consciousness. In fact, the *Prashnopanishad*, which specifically aims at clarifying the nature of creation, explains that, "Prana springs from the atman and is as inseparable from the self as the shadow is from he who casts the shadow." (Ch. 3)

Even the Bible implies that man was given consciousness and life through the breath: "The Lord God formed man out of the dust of the ground and breathing into his nostrils the breath of life, he became a living soul." (Gen. 2:10) This is a symbolic expression of the process of materialization of matter and life together through prana and consciousness. 'Dust' is symbolic of matter and 'blowing the life' means the emergence of prana in matter. The breath itself, being imparted from the cosmic self, contains the cosmic force therein. Thus through the practice of swara yoga, we are attempting to experience the grosser aspect of prana in order to trace it back to its original source.

13

Matter has many stages of existence and manifestation. At one level it is inert. In the process of evolution it manifests life. Later it manifests consciousness, then energy emerges and the final manifestation is knowledge and experience. This is the truth about both physics and metaphysics, about science, tantra and swara yoga.

Energy in matter

According to swara yoga the body is a storehouse of vital energy, a dynamo with infinite electrical currents flowing throughout. The ordinary man sees this body as a combination of flesh, blood and bone. But the yogis and scientists have perceived a greater force behind the physical elements, and that is the force of energy or prana. The prana which motivates the body of man is more subtle than the nucleus of an atom and technology has not yet been able to harness it.

Most people consider the pranic system within the body to be purely physiological, but scientific investigations are coming closer to the truth of swara yoga. Researchers are discovering what the yogis found, that there is an energy link between the physical and psychic bodies. Furthermore, they have arrived at the conclusion that energy or pranic force is convertible into material force and that material force is convertible into pranic force. You know the famous equation of Albert Einstein, $E=mc^2$, that matter is energy in its potential state. This is an ancient truth contained in the Vedas.

There is a small scientific experiment we can use to illustrate this more clearly. If you look at a piece of bone with your naked eye, all you see is a bone. But if you look at a piece of bone under a super microscope, what do you see? First you see living cells, then molecules, then atoms, and later the nucleus of the atom. Ultimately you discover the fantastic behaviour of energy. The piece of bone which appeared to be lifeless matter was not really dead at all, only your eyes were incapable of detecting the living energy within. Therefore, we utilize the practices of swara yoga to make our perception subtle enough to perceive this inherent energy.

Now, even scientists who have gone into the study of energy fields maintain that so-called motionless matter is also permeated with this subtle energy. Therefore prana not only means life, it means existence as well. Where mobility and stability are combined, there is prana. If an object is devoid of prana, it will disintegrate. So science has come to the conclusion that every existing thing is a composite structure of energy and matter. Swara yoga is a means to develop deeper understanding of our own energy structure and to know how to keep it functioning harmoniously.

Photographing the vital energy

Modern science has come across an important discovery which seems to have shown that the energy in the body emits an aura of light. The Vedas clearly state that every object has a pranic field which appears as an encompassing mass of light. In early paintings of great saints, sadhus and gurus, an aura often surrounds the head and sometimes the hands. Some call this light a halo and it can be seen in pictures of Rama, Krishna, Christ, Mohammed, Zarathustra and others. Before the advance of modern science, it was thought that this was created by the imagination of the artist. But the halo or aura is not imaginary, nor is it only peculiar to great and evolved saints.

With the aid of modern scientific equipment, such as Kirlian photography, researchers have shown an aura like an electromagnetic field which can be measured and photographed. Measurements of the changing frequency and amplitude of the electronic field seem to confirm observation of the activities and changing colours of the aura.[1] This is very significant to swara yoga because it correlates with the varying pranic fields emanating from the body and how prana manifests in the body in particular colours depending on the frequency of vibration. By testing people with this

15

equipment the Kirlians have found that every living being has an aura. This aura does not indicate the degree of spiritual attainment, although it is definitely expanded by higher aspirations and sattwic qualities. Even a criminal has an aura, and a murderer or thief can be detected by his specific type of aura and pranic emanations.

Some people have the capacity of mind to perceive and see the aura. They can read it through a subtle faculty of mind. It requires a certain angle of perception and state of mind which can be developed. Swara yoga specifically develops this subtlety of mind and it starts by making the practitioner aware of the pranic vibration in the body and breath.

Kirlian photography and prana

One of the major scientific discoveries which brought the subject of prana to public awareness, as we have already mentioned, was Kirlian photography. The inventors, a husband and wife team called the Kirlians, came across the phenomena in 1939, and since then researchers have been photographing many different types of objects. They found that all life forms emit a particular aura, and that insentient objects can also have an aura for some time. This is relevant to swara yoga, especially as it involves concentration on certain symbols to enable one to perceive the pranic flow in the body.

Hundreds of experiments have been done in Kirlian photography to show differences in auras, for example, in coins held by different people, or in leaves that have fallen naturally and those cut down by a knife. Photographs were made of the thumbs of different people who were healthy and unhealthy, depressed and elated, etc. Separate photographs were taken of a man's hand and a woman's hand and then again when they held hands. It was found that the man's aura had contracted while the woman's had expanded. Experiments have brought researchers to the conclusion that the aura, or electromagnetic radiation of the body, is constantly changing. It can expand and diminish, and it can influence as well as be influenced by others.

In swara yoga the same conclusions were also reached. Here it says that our thoughts and state of mind influence our pranic rhythms, which is what researchers in Kirlian photography also found in relation to the aura. According to one's mental and emotional responses, the aura expands or contracts.[2] For example, when a person is calm and relaxed, the pranic emanations are steady and elongated. But when the person becomes anxious, the aura becomes flared and jagged. After arousing different emotions and thoughts at will, Kirlian photographs showed that the aura automatically changes. By concentrating on the aura itself, it can also be altered. Similarly, by concentrating on his prana, the swara yogi changes the active flow at will.

Researchers also observed that just before death the aura completely vanishes. In swara yoga it is said that when there is no longer any indication of prana, death will ensue. There is a practice whereby the adept can predict death or sickness by gazing at his shadow and then looking into the sky where he can see a duplicate form of the shadow. If there is no reflection in the sky, death can be expected, and if only some areas are reflected, sickness. This is because just before death the pranas and electromagnetic fields withdraw, and therefore the aura diminishes. At the time of death there is no prana, no aura and no life.

So the swara yogis devised different practices to increase the pranic capacity and pranic field or aura. These practices enable us to perceive the subtlety of our existence in relation to the universe. Prana is the basis of life, and in swara yoga we develop the conscious capacity to control it and see that it is not wasted.

3

Ions and
Electromagnetic Fields

During the last half of the twentieth century scientists
have been investigating pranic phenomena and finally
they seem to have come up with a feasible explanation. Just
as yoga talks about the universal prana which permeates
the entire creation, modern scientists have discovered the
same presence of electromagnetic energy. Investigations
show that the atmosphere is charged with electromagnetic
energy which is vital to the preservation of life. Yoga states
that where there is life, there is prana; and what science
has found is that wherever there is life, there are electrical
properties.[1]

In yogic texts prana is equated with lightning, thus
implying that its properties have some similarity to electrical
energy. Prana is also described as being magnetic as it
has positive and negative aspects. Therefore, in order to
understand the basis of swara yoga, it is useful to discuss a
little about the nature of electromagnetic fields.

A living magnet
Scientific investigations have brought modern science and
man closer to yoga. Swara yoga talks of the positive and
negative energy currents flowing in the body, and science has
proven the existence of these flows, which are furthermore
influenced by the ions and the electromagnetic field in the
atmosphere.[2]

18

The electromagnetic energy which surrounds the earth makes it appear to be a gigantic magnet, the north pole being positive and the south pole negative. Each pole attracts opposite and repels like electromagnetic particles, thus creating energy circuits around the terrestrial plane. The particular movements of these electromagnetic currents affect the energy balance in every form of life. Furthermore, the cycle of these currents greatly affects our entire being, and the particular nature of the charged particles influences the different mental and physical processes.

Swara yoga explains this a little more deeply. Here the body is also considered as a living magnet. The head is the positive pole and the feet are the negative pole. To be more precise, we can say that the energy currents circulate specifically in the region of the spinal column, the base of the spine being the negative pole and the top the positive. This magnetic field creates a constant flow of energies between the two poles in an attempt to equalize the energy circuits. In fact, many people even say that you should not sleep with the head towards the west, because the circulation of energy must flow with the earth's energy field.

Though the external influence of energy and prana affects the internal structure, the practices of swara yoga regulate the inner pranic mechanisms, enabling them to function harmoniously irrespective of the outer conditions. Today science is proving this in experiments to control the bioelectromagnetic fields.[3]

Science is only now beginning to view the human organism in the light of a living transmitter of energy. The brain and central nervous system in particular have been seen to act as transmitters and receptors of electromagnetic waves, receiving external information and sending internal information back into the cosmos.[4] Just the simple process of the heart beat sends out a wave of 1–3 cycles per second. So you can imagine how much subtle transfer of energy is going on constantly between you and the cosmos. Therefore, it is of great importance to maintain harmony and equilibrium in our inner and outer environment. The sadhaka practises not only for himself but in order to raise the energy throughout the atmosphere.

Investigating the energy field

When researchers examined the nature and flow of electromagnetic fields, they found they were made up of positively and negatively charged particles called ions, which are so microscopic they can interpenetrate the earth, air and everything. The positive or negative charge of ions in the body has also been seen to influence specific physical and mental functions.[5] Therefore, if you can control these energies, you can control the body and mind.

A predominance of negative ions has been observed to have a stimulating and vitalizing effect on the body, whereas a predominance of positive ions depresses the system.[6] For example, when people are exposed to an excess of positive ions, they become lethargic and if there is constant stimulus, then irritation, headaches and respiratory defects can also develop. When negative ions are again increased, the whole system is revitalized and reactivated.[7] It has been found that ionic charges are essential to the atmosphere and to life. If they are absent, not one creature will survive.

The presence of positive and negative ions in the system ultimately affects the entire body mechanism. They influence the nervous system, rate of respiration, digestion and regulation of the endocrine system,[8] which in turn influences the way we think and respond to certain situations in life. Therefore, the absorption of positive and negative ions in the air we breathe is an important function of the respiratory system. So swara yoga regards breathing as an electrifying experience.

In search of negative ions and prana

When you leave the city and all its industrial complexes and go to a hill station, forest, seaside or river, you always feel invigorated. This is due to the natural abundance of negative ions that cluster in the atmosphere of such regions. When we say 'breath of fresh air', what we really mean is breath of negative ions. Fresh air in the city may contain an abundance of positive ions, so even a breath of fresh air there won't make you feel refreshed. Modern technology is recklessly destroying the natural balance of ions in the atmosphere, especially in more populated areas. Deficiency of negative ions is a major contributing factor to the rise of physical and mental depression people are suffering today. When the mind and body are depressed, how can you expect to live or think correctly? Therefore, in swara yoga or any yoga the sadhaka is advised to breathe pure air and live in a simple environment in order to come closer to the Self.

4

The Nose

GATEWAY TO THE INNER WORLD

In the process of breathing, absorbing prana and circulating energy, the nose plays a vital role. It is an important junction of energy communication between the external and internal worlds. When the external air comes into contact with the nasal passages, minute nerve detectors situated in the mucous membrane of the nose relay impulses to the brain and energy circuits. Swara yoga claims that by manipulation of the breath flowing in and out through the nose you can regulate the inner body mechanisms and develop complete control over all pranic and mental activities.

Scientific investigations have shown that many autonomic and voluntary functions are related to the breath and these nerve components situated at the base of the nose. In fact, it has been reported that the nerves in the nasal mucosa are connected with the visceral, excretory and reproductive organs. Improper breathing and irregularity of the breath in the nostrils can create a disturbance in any of these organs and vice versa.[1] In the *Hatha Yoga Pradipika* it is said that, "Hiccups, asthma, coughing, pain in the head, ears, eyes and other related diseases are generated by disturbance of the breath." (2:17)

It has even been seen that obstruction of the nasal passage can slow down the heart rate and blood circulation, thereby preventing proper tissue oxidation. Further complications are alteration of the flow of lymphatic fluid and disturbance of the alkaline base reserve in the blood and cellular tissues, leading to a concentration of chloride and calcium.[2] It is interesting to note that the proportion of autonomic nerve fibres in the nasal cavity is said to be twenty times greater than in the other parts of the central nervous system. Therefore, the nose has been described as a 'peripheral organ of the autonomic nervous system'.[3]

What we breathe and how we breathe affects our emotions and vice versa. The *Hatha Yoga Pradipika* similarly states that "when breathing is disturbed, the mind also becomes disturbed. Control of the breath enables steadiness of mind." (2:2)

The smell brain
Associated with the faculty of breathing is the sense of smell. When we speak of the nose and its functions, this is another important aspect to be considered. Nervous impulses activated by chemical odours are sent from the nose to the limbic system, a part of the midbrain which transforms perception into cognitive experience. This centre also regulates our emotional responses to the external environment.[4] We are usually unaware of this process unless there happens to be some obvious and potent odour nearby. The sense of smell functions at a non-verbal and subliminal level.

When the sense of smell is triggered off by an actual chemical odour, certain impulses are sent to the olfactory nerve and the rhinencephalon, the centre which stimulates instinctive responses of fear, aggression, pain and particularly sexual behaviour. In fact, in most primitive vertebrates the brain registers the majority of information by smell. Thus the rhinencephalon is known as the 'smell brain'. Smell activates many of our natural and spontaneous reactions, but because we also have higher faculties of awareness and intellect, its influence is far less than in other primates.

Nevertheless, it has been found that the influence of particular chemical odours can create certain emotional reactions within the human body. The smell of a person or

23

an object will determine our reactions and responses to it. Women in particular have been found to be most sensitive to smell, especially during the time of the mid-menstrual cycle.[5] This fact has led science to discover the connection between the sense of smell and the production of sex hormones.

According to tantra, the sense of smell is also connected to mooladhara chakra, the energy centre situated at the base of the spinal column. This centre is the seat of man's spiritual energy. In order to awaken mooladhara, we therefore utilize the yogic practice of concentration in which you gaze at the nosetip. This arouses the sensation of psychic odours, and is particularly associated with that of sandalwood. Different odours stimulate different energy centres, and sandalwood is said to activate the centre at the bottom of the spine. It is also the smell of the subtle body. So even though this practice is based on a physiological process, it enables the awareness to become more sensitive to subtle vibrations. It can even help bring about the awakening of kundalini, the high-powered generator which illumines the hitherto unexplored areas of the brain responsible for all of man's ingenuity, higher knowledge and self-realization.

The nasal circuit
Swara yoga explains that the two major energy circuits, ida and pingala, can be regulated and controlled by means of the breath. If these currents are not flowing properly, it becomes quite evident in the breath. Electro-nasographic research has, in fact, shown charges of electrical potential emitted from the nasal mucous membrane and these charges are generally unequal.[6] It is believed that these charges alter in relation to one's psychophysiological state. In direct connection with swara yoga, we can say there seems to be a relationship between the air passing through the left nostril and electromagnetic currents passing along the left side of the vertebral column and, conversely, the relationship between breathing through the right nostril

and electromagnetic currents passing along the right side of the vertebral column. This is very important in swara yoga because ida, the negative channel, emanates and terminates on the left side, and has greater control over the left half of the body. Conversely, pingala, the positive channel, emanates and terminates on the right side and its influence is greater on the right half of the body. So if there is disturbance in the rhythm or cycles of the breath, there is likely to be some imbalance in the whole body system.

In swara yoga it has been seen that ida and pingala operate alternately and that they flow in a rhythmic cycle. Researchers have noticed that specific hormonal cycles and biorhythms can be detected by changes in the mucosal lining of the nose.[7] Therefore, in order to maintain balance, harmony and equilibrium of body, mind and prana, the *Hatha Yoga Pradipika* states: "If the air is inhaled through the left nostril, it should be expelled again through the right. Then breathing in through the right and retaining, it should be expelled through the left."(2:10) This particular practice, which is known as nadi shodhana, brings about regularity in the whole system and is extremely important in swara yoga for harmonizing the pranic flow.

5

Consciousness in Relation to Energy

In swara yoga the aim is not only to regulate and control the vital and mental capacities through control of the breath. In fact, swara yoga says that by concentrating on the pranic flow, one can experience the existence of supreme consciousness. So far we have discussed prana or Shakti, but how does this relate to consciousness or Shiva? In its primordial state consciousness is united with prana like water and salt in the ocean. When they become separated, they play different roles in the various realms of creation. Shiva is consciousness, and it manifests as mind. Shakti is energy manifesting as prana, and in swara yoga it becomes the tool for understanding consciousness. Just as prana exists in cosmic and individual states, so does consciousness.

Equation of relativity

Tantra and yoga define matter as a gross form of energy. Of course, the energy inherent in matter can be liberated, but still it will not be the final product. Inherent in energy is consciousness. The difference between these three states is only the vibrational rate and density of energy. At the highest and most subtle level of vibration, energy manifests as pure consciousness. As the rate of vibration decreases, it appears to be pure energy, and finally it solidifies into matter. In the reverse order, matter can be transformed into energy, and energy into consciousness. The objective of swara yoga is to experience the inherent energy in matter and mind so that consciousness manifests.

We think the physical body or the mass of the earth, sun, moon and stars are just gross matter because our perception is so limited. In the ultimate analysis, however, all the great scientists and seers found that matter is but one state of energy. In another state of manifestation, matter again becomes prana or light. Yoga applies the same principle to the mind.

The mind is considered as a form of matter which operates at a higher energy level or rate of vibration. The more the mind is absorbed in the physical world, the grosser it becomes and the less the consciousness or awareness can function. This is the dormant or tamasic state of mind. As consciousness and awareness develop, the mind starts to oscillate, to become dynamic or rajasic. Later it becomes completely one-pointed, awakened, and sattwic. By becoming aware of the breath and the flow of prana, you attune the mind to more subtle vibrations. Therefore, swara yoga says first realize the energy potential operating in the body, then realize the potential energy of the mind, and finally realize the inherent consciousness in both.

Consciousness: the primal element

Matter, energy and consciousness are convertible and reconvertible. This is the basic principle of tantra and modern science. Physics defines matter as a combination of trillions of particles, molecules, atoms and subatoms. The difference between each mass is in the arrangement and vibration of the particles. If you change these factors, the mass also changes form.

For example, in a block of ice the particles are closely packed together and vibrate slowly. If you heat the ice, it turns into liquid. The particles move away from each other and begin to vibrate more quickly. When you apply more heat, the water becomes vapour and the particles move further apart, vibrating at greater speed. The ice changes its form but still the basic chemical elements remain the same. Similarly, yoga considers pure consciousness to be the basic element that manifests in the various forms of creation.

It moves, it moves not

Particle physics explains how the atoms of every object interconnect with the particles of the surrounding environment. Thus every manifestation in creation forms part of a never-ending field or matrix of particles. The atoms, electrons, protons, neutrons, photons comprising our bodies, the clothes we wear, the ground on which we walk and the air we breathe are all arranged in different densities, combinations and vibrations, but at a certain point these atoms all interact and interlink. Everything is part of an undifferentiated whole, and whatever exists within this field is changed only by the restructuring of the particles.

In the continual process of nature, all these particles interact and vibrate unceasingly. The field is thus in a state of constant motion, and yet as a whole it is not moving anywhere. This is exactly what is explained in the *Ishopanishad* in reference to the nature of consciousness: "It moves, it moves not. It is far, it is near. It is within all this, and it is outside all this." (mantra 5)

Physics talks about the undifferentiated field, and yoga about an all-pervading consciousness. In reference to this, the greatest scientist of our time, Einstein, has said that, "We may therefore regard matter as being constituted by the regions of space in which the field (consciousness) is extremely intense . . . There is no place in this new kind of physics both for the field (consciousness) and matter, for the field (consciousness) is the only reality."[1]

Cosmic mind and prana

In tantra there is a beautiful concept which explains how the interaction of consciousness with prana manifests as creation. Not only does this apply to cosmic events but to our own personal life as well, because each individual is

28

a complete universe unto himself. Tantra says that before the universe and galaxies came into being, the inherent potential of creation existed in hiranyagarbha, the golden egg or universal womb of creation. This is represented by *bindu*, which means 'point'. It can be likened to a seed with infinite potential. From this tiny point of light, the entire creation unfolds.

Within bindu exist two poles of energy – one positive and the other negative, and at the nucleus is matter. The positive pole represents consciousness or Shiva and can be equated with time. The negative pole represents prana or Shakti and can be equated with space. As long as Shiva and Shakti are together, dormant, there is no movement, no spark, no creation. But as soon as the split takes place and these two forces are separated into positive and negative poles, they begin to interact upon each other. At this point the two poles start to proceed towards each other and eventually they connect at the nucleus.

Time and space have first to be separated before they can meet. When these two forces – time and space, Shiva and Shakti – come together again, a great explosion takes place and the nucleus of matter bursts into trillions of fragments which form the nebulae of creation. These nebulae vibrate at such an incredible speed and velocity that they emanate ultrasonic waves and light. This is the first manifestation of cosmic prana, which is represented by the cosmic body or *virat*. Thus in the process of creation and evolution, we have two definite aspects before us – hiranyagarbha or cosmic mind and virat or cosmic prana.

Swara yoga equates Shakti and Shiva with prana and chitta, which manifest in the body as the two nadis, pingala and ida. In Samkhya philosophy they are known as prakriti and purusha, in Taoism as yin and yang. These are the two forces which uphold the universe and spark off the entire creation.

6

Mind and Consciousness

The ancient yogis were able to define mind and consciousness by becoming receptive to the subtler vibrations in the universe. The more sensitive their awareness became, the more subtle vibrations they were able to perceive. In every realm of existence they perceived the underlying consciousness. The word consciousness has often been confused with the individual mind, but the individual mind is only the tool of consciousness. That capacity which enables us to be aware is more than mind; it is consciousness.

If you dissect the brain, you will not find the mind. It is the instrument of perception. Maybe with the help of modern technology you could detect the prana, but there is no instrument that can measure or calculate the extent of the mind, let alone the inherent quality of consciousness.

Dimensions of the mind

Yoga describes the mind as the creation of *atma shakti* or the creative power of consciousness. In the *Bhagavad Gita* Krishna compares the mind to a chariot, the body and senses to the horses and the atma to the charioteer. These are the three levels from which we operate. In swara yoga each level is associated with a specific nadi. Pingala is responsible for external awareness and motivating the body. Ida withdraws the mind and activates internal awareness. Sushumna is the passage of transcendental consciousness.

30

According to Jung and other modern psychologists, the mind can be categorized into three states – conscious, subconscious and unconscious. In yoga these are termed *jagrit*, *swapna* and *sushupti* respectively. Within these three states, the consciousness undergoes the experiences of mind and body. However, yoga describes a fourth dimension where the finite mind no longer exists. The consciousness travels into a higher dimension called *turiya*, which is beyond objective and subjective experience. There is no individuality, no existence of 'I' and 'you', no past, present or future, only oneness and unity. In this state the individual consciousness and prana return to the cosmic body.

Three states of consciousness
In jagrit, the waking state, the mundane world is perceived through the gross body or *sthula sharira*. The *Mandukyopanishad* says that here "the enjoyment lies in the visible objects of the world". (v. 3) In jagrit there is association with the external world through the five sensory organs, the *jnanendriyas* (the ears, eyes, tongue, nose and skin) and through the five organs of action, the *karmendriyas* (the hands, feet, speech, reproductive and excretory organs). In the waking state information is interpreted by *manas* (thought/counterthought), *buddhi* (discrimination), *ahamkara* (ego) and *chitta* (memory). These are all associated with the functions of pingala nadi.

At a deeper level the consciousness encounters subjective experience in the subconscious realm of swapna, the dream state. Here the experiences are those of the astral or subtle body, the *sukshma sharira*. The consciousness becomes involved in the mental impressions of jagrit, undergoing the memories in the *karmashaya*, the place where every action, thought and word is stored. In the subconscious there is no objective experience through the senses. The experiences are purely mental and therefore it is associated with ida nadi.

When the unconscious layer of the mind is entered, one undergoes the experiences of the causal or etheric body, the

31

karana sharira. This is sushupti, described in the *Manduk-yopanishad* as the realm of "dreamless sleep, lying beyond desire in the territory of intuition". (v. 5) Here the gross and subtle minds no longer function; "they are absorbed in the self" and the consciousness is not bound by time or space. Nevertheless, there remains a trace of individual existence and "the atman is still caught in darkness". The unconscious realm is associated with sushumna nadi before it is awakened. Only when it is fully illumined can we experience the reality of consciousness.

Throughout life we are continually undergoing these three states of consciousness without retaining any awareness of the experiences. However, the yogis of old found that by maintaining undivided attention on the movement of the breath and prana, they could pass from one state to the next without losing awareness. They could even pass beyond the barriers of the finite mind into the infinite. It is written in *Mandukyopanishad* that then the atma "remains oblivious to the external, intermediate and internal worlds, and enters into turiya, where neither sight nor thought can penetrate." (v. 7) In fact, turiya cannot be described in terms of the empirical world because there are no poles of duality. Individual consciousness unites with its source, or pure atman.

When the consciousness is absorbed in jagrit, awareness of swapna and sushupti is not there. In swapna nothing exists except that reality, and the same applies to sushupti. But all these levels of mind can be experienced simultaneously, and the purpose of yoga is to awaken our awareness of each state and thereby bring the mind closer together. We live under the dominion of duality, ida and pingala. While they control the body and mind, the consciousness has to undergo those experiences. Swara yoga aims to bring about a balance between ida and pingala duality, and thus awaken sushumna, or the pure consciousness.

Who am I?

Change in the state of consciousness is brought about by various physical and subtle factors. The difference between one state and another can more readily be seen from a physiological level. Neurologists have shown that the pains and pleasures we experience in each state are just the play of the brain chemistry, so how can we say which level of experience is reality? It is difficult to know, for example, whether waking or dreaming is the real experience, and whether this conscious reality is what we are or if the subconscious and unconscious are the real states of existence from which all the other states manifest. In swara yoga it is said that if you absorb your concentration in the breath and prana, you realize that you are the breath and the body is the manifestation of that breath and consciousness. So the question arises – 'Who am I?'

At the conscious level the physical body and mind are the reality, but at another level they cease to exist, and you become something else, so you cannot say that you are the mind and body alone. It is like the story of Chuang-tzu, who dreamt he was a butterfly. When he woke up he asked, "Am I a man dreaming I am a butterfly or a butterfly dreaming I am a man?" The mind and consciousness can take any shape, which becomes reality in that moment. Therefore, swara yoga says to realize the true identity of the consciousness in its pure form as atma.

Modern science, psychology and neurochemistry may have discovered the chemical reactions which alter our states of consciousness, but they cannot define precisely what consciousness is. They cannot explain the process where the consciousness can be set free from the limitations of individuality. So far only yoga has been able to solve the problem with its systematic techniques of developing our awareness through subtler realms of consciousness. In its true essence the consciousness has no mind or body other than its pure and cosmic form.

7

Sound and Form of the Swara

In swara yoga the function of the breath is very scientific. When the awareness is absorbed in the breath, in its movement, in its sound, it becomes the vehicle for traversing the superficial layers of the mind and attaining higher experiences beyond the influence of the external senses.

Yoga and tantra explain that the breath vibrates with the force of prana. Vibrations cannot exist without creating a sound frequency. Therefore, the breath also has a specific sound which is heard at a particular level of consciousness. In the *Yoga Chudamani Upanishad* it is explained that, "The breath goes out making the sound of Ham and comes in producing the sound So, whereby the jiva continually repeats the mantra Ham-So 21,600 times every twenty-four hours. This continual repetition of the mantra is known as ajapa japa." (v. 31–32)

The Upanishads further state that by conscious mental repetition of the mantra So-Ham with the breath, the mantra manifests as an audible sound in the inner ear. On hearing this, one becomes freed from karma and samskara. To investigate this claim, we will have to experience the mantra of the breath and we will have to experience its effect at the different levels of mind and consciousness.

Dimensions of sound

The sound we hear with the ears and the faculty of the brain is only one level of perception. If sound waves exist at the conscious level, they must also exist at the subtler levels. The human ear has a very limited range of perception. We know that cats, dolphins, bats and many other animals have such an acute sense of hearing that they can perceive frequencies inaudible to the human ear. As the frequency becomes higher, our ears fail to pick up the vibrations, although the sound is still there. In the same way, although we do not hear the subtler sound of the breath, it creates sound waves in the deeper realms of our consciousness.

As the breath becomes finer, the sound frequencies become more intense and subtle. In this way, they are heard internally from the subconscious realm, then the unconscious and finally the superconscious where sound becomes transcendental. Normally we are unable to perceive the existence of sound in those realms because we are unaware of those parts of our mind. Those centres of our brain are not active. But when we can experience the subconscious area of the mind with awareness, then the sounds manifesting in that realm also become audible. The same principle applies in regard to unconscious and transcendental vibrations.

The ancient rishis and yogis who had contacted deeper layers of the mind through meditation perceived the sounds of subtler vibrations. Before entering the transcendental state, they heard the sound of the outgoing and ingoing breath, the sound of Ham-So-Ham-So-Ham . . .

Sound also exists in the dimension of turiya, but then there is no individual mind to perceive it. That is the sound of the vibration of the universe, the vibration of Om. In the unconscious realm there is the sound of Ham-So. When you remove the individuality of the finite mind, the 'veil' between Ham (Shakti – the individual jiva) and So (Shiva – cosmic consciousness) is lifted. The sound of the breath is the direct link between the lower and higher experience.

Mantra of the breath

When we speak of mantra in relation to the breath, what does it actually signify? A mantra is more than a sound vibration. The word mantra is made up of two roots: *man*, which means contemplation, and *tra*, which means to liberate. When the transcendental sound of the breath is repeatedly perceived, the consciousness becomes liberated or freed from the finite mind. The mantra of the breath releases the inherent energies required for this liberation. This is not religious terminology, it is purely scientific.

The root *man* also means reflection (*manana*). Mantra brings liberation through reflection, and the same process takes place in regard to the breath. By reflection on the sound of the breath, it becomes realized and the mind becomes absorbed in that manifestation. When this happens, the consciousness in no longer bound to the sensual world. It becomes one with the sound vibration at deeper levels of mind.

Yantra of the breath

The Upanishads declare that liberation of consciousness from mind is freedom from samskara and karma. So, what is this relationship between the mind and karma?

Every experience of the five organs of sense and the five organs of action is stored in the subconscious and unconscious mind in a particular geometrical form known as a *yantra* or archetype. When you see an object or smell an odour, when something makes you happy or sad, the memory of that experience is stored in symbolic form, which represents the whole experience. It is similar to the DNA molecule, which is a complete representation of the entire genetic makeup. In the same way, every experience in your life is recorded in a specific symbolic form called a yantra. Thus the mantra of the breath is the sound vibration and the yantra is the form.

Repetition of the mantra with the breath brings the mind into the subconscious level and then it goes deeper into the unconscious. When the consciousness is absorbed in the deeper realms of the mind and there are no external distractions, then the yantra of the breath manifests and

36

becomes a living experience. Reflection on the yantra is therefore the process of concentrating the mind until it arrives at the final point of illumination.

On reaching that point of concentration where the yantra becomes manifest, an explosion of energy occurs. The same thing is explained in the tantras, where it is stated that the two poles of relativity, Shiva and Shakti, time and space, come together and meet in the nucleus. Then creation bursts forth into existence! Hence, you could even say that concentration on the breath's yantra subsequently leads to what people call a 'mind blowing experience'.

Concentration of mind

Concentrating on the mantra or yantra of the breath is one of the most powerful methods of introverting the restless mind. The process of concentration has four stages: introversion (*pratyahara*), concentration (*dharana*), meditation (*dhyana*) and finally transcendence (*samadhi*). These four distinct stages represent the distances between the two aspects or poles of the mind and perception.

The word concentration implies one-pointedness which increases in strength by the contraction of volume. In the practice of concentration this is what happens to the mind. During pratyahara the two poles of time and space begin to separate from normal conscious perception. In dharana they reach their opposite position. In dhyana they begin to move closer together and in samadhi they meet again at the nucleus. Then the explosion takes place and awareness of the mantra is left behind in the reality of the finite mind. Thus consciousness breaks out of the limited, individual experience represented by So-Ham into the cosmic experience of Om.

8

The Koshas

For millennia yogis have been saying that man's being extends far beyond what the eye can perceive. Of course, everyone is aware of themselves through the capacity to think and cognize. But our existence is far more than matter and intellect. If we were able to experience the body and mind through our subtle eyes, if we could perceive the body behind the body and the mind behind the mind, what would we see?

First of all we would see the underlying energy structure, which gives life to the physical body. Even subtler still we would perceive the whole process being motivated by mind and thought. Behind that mind we would see the operation of a higher type of mind, what we call intuition. And beyond intuition we would experience nothing but the absolute reality of our existence.

The five sheaths

Swara yoga describes man as being composed of five areas of existence, termed the *pancha koshas*. The general translation of *kosha* is sheath, and *pancha* means five. Each kosha is indicative of a particular sphere of existence and *maya* means 'composed of'. *Annamaya kosha*, the first sheath, is composed of *anna* or food. It is the physical body and brain. *Pranamaya kosha*, the second kosha, is composed of prana. *Manomaya kosha*, the third, is composed of *manas* or mind. *Vijnanamaya kosha*, the fourth, is composed of inner knowledge or intuition. *Anandamaya kosha* is the sublime experience of ananda or bliss.   '

Kosha or Body	Psychological Dimension	Physiological State	Experienced as
Annamaya Kosha (food body)	Conscious Mind	Wakeful Awareness	Awareness of physical body
Pranamaya Kosha (pranic body)			Awareness of physiological functions, e.g. digestion, circulation
Manomaya Kosha (mental body)	Subconscious Mind	Dreaming Awareness	Awareness of mental and emotional processes
Vijnanamaya Kosha (intuitive body)			Awareness of psychic and casual dimensions
Anandamaya Kosha (bliss body)	Unconscious Mind to Superconscious Mind	Deep Sleep/ Meditative Awareness	Unconsciousness; Transcendental Awareness

The four categories of mind – conscious, subconscious, unconscious and superconscious, are experienced in the various koshas. Each capacity of mind and body is composed from the material of that kosha.

All the koshas are intricately connected and they continually influence and interact with one another. Pranamaya kosha is the intermediate link between conscious and subconscious. Vijnanamaya kosha is the link between subconscious and unconscious. These five koshas constitute every human being; the physical body is only a fraction of our total range of experience.

In swara yoga, by feeling the physical breath in the nose and acting in accordance with the flow of the swara, you are utilizing the conscious mind and physical body or annamaya kosha. Manipulating the breath and pranic flow and increasing its capacity stimulates pranamaya kosha. The practice of concentration utilizes manomaya kosha. Doing trataka on the tattwa yantras awakens vijnanamaya kosha. But to influence anandamaya kosha there is really no meditation necessary because in this kosha there is only a trace of awareness and no possibility of functioning.

The first stage of swara yoga awakens your awareness of pranamaya kosha, the direct link between mind and body, annamaya and manomaya kosha, and takes you into the subtler reams of existence. Later, the awareness moves into manomaya and vijnanamaya kosha as the practices start to unfold.

Evolution through the koshas
During the different incarnations, the consciousness has been evolving simultaneously with the mental and physical capacities through which it experiences. Here we are not referring to Darwin's theory of the natural evolution of the species and the animal body. Evolution here means the ascent and expansion of consciousness. By means of matter the consciousness evolves and goes beyond. Thus evolution is a process of transformation. In the primal stages, life is dependent on the laws of nature, but once we come into the sphere of human experience a new faculty of conscious awareness opens up. It is this awareness which enables us to speed up the process of our evolution. Swara yoga is very important in this process because it enables us to enter the higher realms of vibration much more quickly.

In the course of time, matter evolves into energy and then into pure consciousness. Energy is the evolved form of matter. It is a slow, continual process as far as the natural evolution of the human body is concerned. Millions of years ago the human form was virtually the same as it is today.

40

We may have been a little taller, shorter, fatter or thinner, depending on environmental conditions. Of course, the human brain was much smaller then, but still it has not yet fully evolved because, as we know, only a minute portion of it is in conscious operation, the other nine-tenths are waiting to be awakened.

It is a physiological fact that the instinctive portion of the brain is in constant use, whereas the higher frontal region is seldom used. It is the purpose of swara yoga to activate these dormant centres. In terms of evolution, our minds are still absorbed in annamaya kosha, the realm of matter. But the higher brain centres penetrate into the subtler koshas. So far, science knows little about the 'silent areas' or the brain and is only just becoming aware of all the different realms in which it can function.

Man has to activate the remaining nine-tenths of his brain, there is no doubt about it. This is the process of evolution, and it can only be accelerated by a scientific system. Total transformation can take place in one lifetime if one is regular in one's practice of yoga. Just as matter is artificially turned into gas by applying heat, the gross mind can be transformed into pure consciousness by the 'fire of yoga'.

The techniques of yoga restructure the internal body system so that prana can flow freely without blockages. The quantum of prana has to be increased so that it becomes powerful and vital. Only in this way can we awaken the dormant areas of the brain. This is where swara yoga becomes essential.

Evolution is the ascendance of individual awareness from the material realm to the subtler and higher levels of existence where the mind becomes conscious and extends itself from annamaya kosha to vijnanamaya or even anandamaya kosha. This is the aim of swara yoga, nothing else. Therefore, we have to understand this science of the ancient rishis, interpret it correctly and integrate it into our daily lives, so that we too can share in their realizations.

9

The Prana Vayus

While studying the breath, the swara yogis noticed that it produced specific energy waves throughout the body. They saw how prana is circulated in the various regions of the body through the medium of the breath. And they found that as prana circulates, it is modified and adapted to the functions of each particular organ and region. According to these different modifications of prana, the *prana vayus* or pranic airs were classified.

In the *Prashnopanishad* it is explained that the "chief prana allots functions to the lower pranas in the same way as an emperor posts his officials in different parts of his domain". In all, there are ten vayus, and of these five are said to have greater influence on the body. They are known as the *pancha pranas*: prana, apana, samana, udana and vyana. The five remaining vayus, having less potential, are called *upa pranas* or subsidiary pranas.

All the vayus are comprised of the jiva's prana, not the pure maha prana. In the *Kaushitaki Upanishad* it is described how "each sense has its own prana, which stems from the one prana".

The body as well as the faculties of the mind and senses are all connected directly with the prana vayu. In the *Prashnopanishad* it is told how the senses and the mind once claimed themselves to be the 'rulers' of the body. But prana reproved them saying, "Don't be deluded. It is I alone, dividing myself fivefold, who support and keep the body intact." Having said this, prana withdrew from the body. The mind and senses also found themselves withdrawn from the body "just as bees leave the hive when the queen departs and return when she returns". (2:2–4) It is the maha prana which is responsible for our every thought and action, while it is the prana vayus which carry them out.

Prana, apana and samana
Each vayu is located in a different region of the body according to its particular direction of flow. The most powerful are prana and apana, the upward and downward movements. Prana vayu functions in the thoracic region to stimulate the respiratory system and the absorption of prana. When the muscle known as the diaphragm contracts, a vacuum is created in the lungs which sucks in air. It is therefore known as the 'in breath'.

Working in opposition to this function is apana, the 'out breath', which is located below the navel in the pelvic region. It is the energy of expulsion, which is stimulated in the lower intestines and urinary/excretory complex. The downward action of apana eliminates wind and excreta from the body.

The whole body is ruled by these two movements of prana and apana. During the day, the action of prana predominates and at night it becomes subservient to apana. The *Dhyana Bindu Upanishad* says that because of prana and apana the *jiva* or individual soul oscillates up and down, caught in the snare of two opposite moving forces and bound by duality. The jiva is compared to a bird which, tied to its perch, flies away but is pulled back again.

However, the key to liberation lies in samana, the third vayu, which equalizes prana and apana. Samana is the 'middle breath' located between the heart and the navel, and its main function is assimilating prana. Physiologically it generates vitality in the liver, pancreas, stomach and digestive tract. In the process of breathing, samana is the time gap between inhalation and exhalation.

43

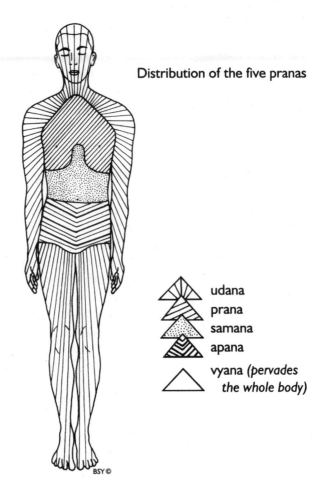

Distribution of the five pranas

udana
prana
samana
apana
vyana (*pervades the whole body*)

Samana links prana and apana, making their movements complementary rather than opposed. When the assimilation and storage of prana is increased, the vital capacity is strengthened. Thus the *Brihadaranyaka Upanishad* states that death does not come to one who increases the middle breath. Therefore, the yogis devised the practice of kumbhaka or breath retention in order to increase the time gap between inhalation and exhalation, thereby uniting prana and apana with samana.

44

Yoga is only accomplished when the natural movements of prana and apana are reversed so that apana moves up and prana moves down, and they unite with samana in the navel centre. The meeting of the two opposite energies generates an incredible force and pushes prana through sushumna nadi, thus awakening the entire pranic capacity, raising the consciousness and enlightening the soul. So, in samana we have the tantric principle of two opposite forces, one negative, the other positive, being brought together in order to explode the creative potential of the nucleus.

Udana, vyana and the upa pranas
After the middle breath another vayu action occurs, udana, which is said by the *Maitri Upanishad* to "bring up and carry down what has been eaten". Udana is called the 'up breath' and is specifically located in the throat and face enabling swallowing, facial expression and speech. It is also responsible for maintaining the strength in every muscle. When prana and apana unite with samana, it is udana which moves up and finally "passes through the tenth gate (sahasrara chakra) towards the higher worlds".

Under normal circumstances udana carries prana from samana to the fifth vayu, vyana. Vyana spreads prana throughout the whole body, regulating and circulating food nutrients, fluids and energy. It holds all the parts of the body together and resists disintegration of the body. When prana moves, it is followed by samana, both creating apana, assisted by udana. The four actions produce vyana, but at the same time they cannot exist without the presence of vyana. Thus these five pranas are very intricately linked. It is said that at the time of death, when prana involutes upon itself, the vital functions of the mind and senses, which represent aspects of the pranic expressions, all withdraw into vyana. It means all the pranas are interdependent but integrated by vyana.

The actions of these five pranas give rise to five upa pranas, which add the 'finishing touches' to the body

45

mechanisms. The eyes are lubricated and kept clean by the blinking power of *kurma*. *Krikara* stimulates hunger, thirst, sneezing and coughing. *Devadatta* induces sleep and yawning, and *naga* hiccup and belching. Finally, after death *dhananjaya* lingers with the remnants of the body.

The pranic body

If we could see the movements of prana vayu, we would perceive the pranic body. Sometimes when a person dies other people imagine they see a ghost, but in actual fact they are seeing that prana which is leaving the body, and this is not something supernatural which has to be feared.

Physics describes a subtle field consisting of charged particles that surrounds and takes the shape of the physical body. This field can be influenced by the internal organs and mental activities and also by the external electric and magnetic fields. We can say it is possibly the grosser manifestation of prana.

The pranic body is a network of flowing energy in the shape of the physical body, but radiating outward just as light emanates beyond the bulb. Its form is not static; it expands and contracts. Decrease in the vital capacity of any vayu causes contraction of the pranic body, while increase causes expansion. The mind and emotions also utilize prana and the pranic body is greatly influenced by states of mind. Negative thoughts lower the prana and exhaust your mind whereas positive thoughts enhance the prana and frame of mind.

In fact, the pranic body is affected by our whole way of living and the pranic functions in turn affect our capacities and attitudes in life. Through the practice of swara yoga we become aware of the mutual interaction between prana and mind and learn to live and work in coordination with the pranas rather than against them.

To be able to move the awareness into the pranic body is to come one step closer to the ultimate reality. The *Kaushitaki Upanishad* states: "It is prana alone as the

46

conscious self that breathes life into this body. Prana is the essence of the life breath. And what is the life breath? It is pure consciousness. And what is pure consciousness? It is the life breath." (v. 3)

10

Nadis

The presence of positively and negatively charged particles activating the body and mind enables us to live in this world, but nature's wonders do not stop there. Man has devised a method to split the atom and release nuclear energy. In the same way he can also release a greater quantum of energy within his own being. In ancient days rishis used their knowledge of the principles of nature to boost the pranic energy in order to accelerate the evolution of human consciousness. The only difference between modern and ancient methods of producing energy is that one utilizes external sources and the other internal.

The pranic network within the body operates on much the same basis as the energy system in nuclear, hydraulic and thermal power stations. The pressure of rapidly flowing water or rising steam rotates turbines which generate electricity. This action can create a powerful magnetic field that can be collected and stored in accumulators. Similarly, yogis describe how the pranic field within the body is charged by respiration. The process of respiration thus generates energy. This energy can then be directed into certain pranic accumulators, known as chakras, for storage.

Accumulation of energy is only a part of the picture; it must then be used efficiently. From the electrical power station, the energy is sent to substations through special high voltage wire cabling. Once it has reached this stage of processing, it is passed through transformers which reduce the voltage so that it is useful for specific purposes. The same principle applies to the physical body, only here the high voltage channels for conduction of energy are not wire cables, they are nadis.

The nadi network

The physical body is structured by an underlying system of nadis. In recent times the nadi system has been associated with the nervous system. However, references in the *Chhandogya* and *Brihadaranyaka Upanishads* clearly state that nadis are entirely subtle in nature. The word *nadi* means flow. The Upanishads explain that the nadis penetrate the body from the soles of the feet to the crown of the head, carrying prana, the breath of life. The atman is the source of shakti and the animator of all the worlds.

The entire network of nadis is so vast that even yogic texts differ in their calculation of the exact number. References in the *Goraksha Sataka* or *Samhita* and *Hatha Yoga Pradipika* place their number at 72,000; the *Prapanchasara Tantra* says 300,000; while the *Shiva Samhita* states that 350,000 emerge from the navel centre. Regardless of the exact figure, the description of their structure is always the same – thin strand-like threads, similar to those of the lotus stem, which emanate from the spinal column.

Scientific research has been carried out to determine what and where nadis are. Dr Hiroshi Motoyama has found stable voltages of electromagnetic currents flowing within close proximity to the nervous system.[1] He takes this as evidence for the existence of nadis and acupuncture meridians.

The major nadis

In any electrical circuit, three specific wires are required for conduction – one positive, one negative and one neutral. Likewise, within the body there are three specific nadis for conducting energy. In yoga we refer to the negative line as *ida*, the channel of manas shakti or mental force. The positive line is *pingala*, which channels the dynamic energy of prana shakti. In order to avoid short-circuiting of these lines there is a third channel, *sushumna*, which functions as an earth wire, being rooted in mooladhara chakra, when it is in its dormant state. But the real purpose of sushumna is to provide a channel for the spiritual energy, which is a greater force than either manas or prana shakti. For this reason the yogis developed particular techniques to activate sushumna.

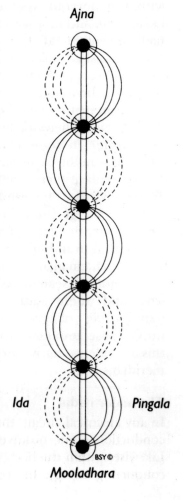

Of all the thousands of nadis, sushumna is said to be the most important. The *Shiva Swarodaya* names ten major nadis which connect to the 'doorways' leading in and out of the body. Of these ten, ida, pingala and sushumna are most important. They are the high voltage wires which conduct the energy to the substations or chakras situated along the spinal column. The seven lesser nadis are: *gandhari*, connected to the left eye; *hastijihva*, connected to the right eye; *poosha*, connected to the right ear; *yashaswini*, connected to the left ear; *alambusha*, connected to the mouth; *kuhu*, connected to the reproductive organs; *shankhini*, connected to the rectum. Other Upanishads talk about 14 to 19 significant nadis and include: *jihva, kurma, payaswini, saraswati, saumya, shura, varuni, vilambha* and *vishvodari*. Little is said about the nature or function of these nadis in swara yoga, so for all practical purposes

Ajna

Ida

Pingala

Mooladhara

50

one need only concentrate on ida, pingala and sushumna, as these three govern the whole system of the nadis and body processes.

Positive and negative aspect

It is necessary to understand that ida and pingala are opposite aspects of the one prana or shakti. At the macrocosmic level, maha prana ranges from gross and tangible to subtle and intangible. Similarly, in the body, microcosmic prana is polarized into ida and pingala, and these are symbolized by the terms negative and positive. These terms are purely descriptive and should not be confused with positive and negative ions or with positive and negative states of mind. For example, the overall effect of negative ions in the body is said to be 'positive', whereas the positive symbolism of pingala refers to the physical level of activation, and the negative symbolism of ida refers to the mental level. Therefore, we have to be careful that we have a clear understanding of positive and negative energy when we talk about the nadis.

Ida pathway

Ida nadi, the negative channel, brings consciousness into every part of the body. The *Shiva Swarodaya* likens its nature to the energy created by the moon; therefore, it is also known as the *chandra* or lunar nadi. Ida is associated with the parasympathetic nervous system (PNS), which sends impulses to the visceral organs to stimulate the internal processes. This creates a general state of relaxation in the superficial muscles, thus lowering the outer body temperature. Therefore, it is said that ida is cooling, relaxing and introverting.

The pathway of ida differs from that of pingala. Ida originates at a point just below the base of the spine where the first energy centre, known as mooladhara chakra, is located. It emerges from the left side of mooladhara and spirals upwards, intersecting at the other four energy centres and plexuses in the spinal column, and comes to a point of termination at the root of the left nostril, which joins ajna chakra, the sixth energy centre.

Some texts describe ida as rising straight up from mooladhara to ajna without intersecting at any junction. This could be taken to be symbolic of the fact that the energy fields of ida govern the left side of the spinal column and the whole left half of the body. In this regard the analogy of the magnet is useful in terms of describing positive and negative poles and their relativity. If we cut a magnet in half, either end of the magnet assumes opposite polarity. Similarly, in the body, organs on the right are polarized so that pingala governs the right side of the organ and ida the left.

According to swara yoga, left nostril breathing influences the activities of manas shakti, and indicates that introversion and mental creativity predominate so that any extremely dynamic or extrovert activity should be avoided. The swara yogi thus manipulates the flow of air in the left nostril in order to control ida directly and either bring about its influence at will or suppress it when necessary.

Pingala pathway

Pingala is the transmitter of prana shakti. It is the positive aspect, also known as the *surya* or solar nadi because its energy is as invigorating as the sun's rays. Pingala energy activates the physical body and externalizes awareness. It is associated with the sympathetic nervous system (SNS), which releases adrenaline to stimulate the superficial muscles. The SNS prepares the body to cope with stress and external activity; for example, it makes the heart beat rapidly and heats the body. Therefore, it is said that pingala is energizing, heating and extroverting.

Pingala emerges on the right hand side of mooladhara, exactly opposite to ida. It spirals up the spinal column, crossing ida at the four major energy centres, and terminates at the root of the right nostril. Pingala governs the whole right side of the body. To control pingala the breath in the right nostril is manipulated.

Right and left hemispheres of the brain

The specific functions of the cerebral region of the brain also correlate with the activities of ida and pingala. The cerebrum is symmetrical, consisting of the right and left hemispheres. The right hemisphere governs the left side of the body and the left hemisphere governs the right side of the body. Ida is connected to the right hemisphere and pingala to the left.

The right hemisphere processes information in a diffuse and wholistic manner. It controls orientation in space and is particularly sensitive to the vibrational realm of existence and those experiences which are intangible to the external sense receptors. Thus it is responsible for psychic and extrasensory perception, and stimulates creative, artistic and musical abilities. Conversely, the left hemisphere in relation to pingala is responsible for rational, analytical and mathematical ability. In the left hemisphere, information is processed sequentially, linearly and logically.[2] In this way the hemispheres, in association with the nadis, control and motivate our responses in day to day life.

Each hemisphere is also associated with the arousal of different emotions. Some neurologists have described the right hemisphere as 'sad' and the left as 'happy'.[3] It has even been observed that a positive emotional stimulus activates the left hemisphere and a negative emotional stimulus stimulates the right. Furthermore, left/right activities cause a person to react in a particular manner under certain circumstances.[4] The left hemisphere has been noted to create an aggressive response or the 'fight' reaction, whereas the right hemisphere causes a person to withdraw and become a passive participant or to 'flee'.

Neurologists have also found a correlation between male/female responses and left/right brain functions. It seems that women are liable to rely more on right hemisphere strategies than men, which verifies why they are considered to be ida predominant. As far as science has probed, the difference in mental capacities is possibly related to different ratios of sex hormones affecting the structure of the brain.[5] Whatever the physiological cause may be, it definitely corresponds to the fact that ida is considered the female principle and pingala the male.

The tantric concept of Shiva/Shakti, the twin forces existing within each individual, can be seen in the structure of the brain and pranic body in terms of ida and pingala. It certainly substantiates the idea of a person having two minds, one positive and the other negative, and even the theory that there is a male and female side in everyone.

11

Triune Energy System

We have seen how the body is divided into two definite divisions or zones according to the flow of energy and magnetic pull of positive and negative forces. However, there is a third aspect yet to be mentioned. In the central axis where the two adjoining sides meet, the positive and negative energies become equalized and create a neutral energy field running straight up and down through the centre. In yoga this important pathway is called sushumna nadi.

Sushumna emerges from the base of the spine, the same as ida and pingala, but without diverging right or left, it travels directly up through the centre, piercing the main chakras and plexuses along the route. Sushumna unites with ida and pingala at ajna chakra in the region of the medulla oblongata. Thus it is considered to correspond with the central or cerebrospinal nervous system (CNS). The CNS carries impulses to the whole system. It is one main system, running from the base of the spine to the brain, and sushumna is also located in the same position.

At man's present stage of evolution sushumna lies dormant. We know that it has tremendous potential, but unless we can apply some particular method to activate it, at the rate we are evolving it will take thousands of years. Therefore, through the manipulation of the swara yogis devised the means of awakening sushumna. Under normal circumstances energy travels up either ida or pingala. However, if both these energies can be brought together, a more powerful force, known as kundalini shakti, will awaken. Kundalini is the spiritual force which operates at very high frequencies. In comparison to the energies of ida and pingala, this force is like a laser beam. However, before kundalini energy is generated, the sushumna passage must first be opened.

When sushumna is active, the breath flows through both nostrils simultaneously. Every hour and twenty minutes after sunrise, the central nadi flows for a few moments. After practising pranayama or when the mind becomes one-pointed, or when one is about to commit some criminal act, sushumna also flows. Therefore, in swara yoga there is a strict warning about it. When sushumna nadi flows, spiritual as well as criminal tendencies can arise.

Both the suicidal terrorist and the yogi in deep meditation have sushumna flowing. When you are about to engage in some sort of crime or assault in battle, sushumna flows. It also flows during the exhilaration one feels after climbing a mountain or in completing an important task, and when sushumna flows the whole brain operates. In ida or pingala only half the brain is active, but in sushumna both the karmendriyas and jnanendriyas, that is the physical organs and the mental organs, function simultaneously and you become very powerful, whether in spiritual or in mundane life.

Nadis within sushumna

The inner structure of sushumna is quite complex. It is not just a hollow tube lying still and lifeless. Sometimes there is a slight flow of energy within the nadi and it becomes slightly activated. This can be detected by the simultaneous flow of air through both nostrils. Of course, it does not mean that kundalini has risen; it only implies that there is activation or opening of sushumna. Ordinarily the impulses created have a very weak charge when compared to the fully awakened

56

state of the adept. Concentration on sushumna in combination with specifically designed yogic practices slowly builds up the charge in preparation for kundalini awakening.

While concentrating on sushumna, three other nadis which lie within the inner walls of sushumna are also brought into operation. The deeper you go, the more refined the nadis become. Just inside the outer surface is *vajra nadi*, within this lies *chitra* or *chitrini nadi*, and deeper still is the subtlest *brahma nadi*. Brahma nadi is so called because it is via this channel that the higher centres of consciousness are directly stimulated. When kundalini shakti passes into this channel, transcendental experiences start to take place.

As long as sushumna is dormant and either ida or pingala is functioning, all the other nadis fall under the positive and negative influences of manas and prana shakti. In order to activate sushumna, the swara yogi manipulates his breath so that it flows evenly through both nostrils for long periods. The *Hatha Yoga Pradipika* explains that "sushumna remains closed owing to the impurities of the nadis". Therefore, we should try to purify the whole system first, and then sushumna will automatically open. Then we must learn to control ida and pingala so that the positive and negative energy flows can be harmonized, thereby creating the perfect condition for activating sushumna.

Symbolism of the triune energy
The negative force of ida, the positive force of pingala and the neutral force of sushumna are present in all forms of creation. These three aspects of energy, in different proportions, enable nature to produce diverse manifestations and the quantum of energy determines the particular characteristics of that form. In swara yoga we begin to see the positive, negative and neutral aspects of the three nadis.

In the following chart, ida is represented by sattwa while sushumna represents tamas. It means that sushumna is in a state of inertia or tamoguna. This is because in the point of evolution prior to awakening, there is no movement in sushumna. However, the nadi contains within itself the three other nadis which represent the three qualities of nature and the potentiality of becoming fully awakened and evolved. Sushumna represents tamas, vajra nadi represents rajas and chitrini nadi represents sattwa. Transcendence of the three gunas, or modes of nature, means evolving beyond time and space, mind and body, ida and pingala. At that point in evolution, the entire shakti travels through brahma nadi, thus transforming the inert nature of sushumna and transcendence of the awareness of individual existence and experience takes place.

Ida	Pingala	Sushumna
chitta	prana	kundalini
mental	vital	supramental
negative	positive	neutral
feminine	masculine	androgynous
yin	yang	tao
moon	sun	light
cold	hot	temperate
intuition	logic	wisdom
desire	action	knowledge
internal	external	centred
night	day	sunset/dawn
passive	dynamic	balanced
subjectivity	objectivity	awareness
parasympathetic	sympathetic	cerebrospinal
Yamuna	Ganga	Saraswati
blue	red	yellow
Brahma	Vishnu	Rudra
subconscious mind	conscious mind	unconscious mind (in dormancy)
sattwa	rajas	tamas
A	U	M

Experience of the swara in sushumna

In swara yoga it is said that if sushumna flows for a very long time, it means your mind is going to transcend the barrier of subject and object, ida and pingala. For the householders, who are engaged in worldly duties, this state may not be desirable, but it is what the yogi is striving for. In India, cases have been witnessed where people were able to predict their time of death several days beforehand by observing the continual flow of sushumna.

So the flowing of sushumna for a long period of time is an indication that one of two things is about to happen. In the case of the yogi, it means you are about to transcend body, mind and the object, and enjoy samadhi. When the awakening of kundalini takes place, the first thing that happens is sushumna becomes charged by the kundalini energy. The whole spinal passage becomes heated, active and full of experiences. In the case of the average person, it means you are going to transcend the body and enjoy life beyond the empirical realm, but the kundalini is not necessarily awakened.

12

Chakras

Within the subtle structure of the pranic network, every nadi has a specific route, and at certain points all the nadis come together to form centres of pranic and psychic energy known as chakras. *Chakra* is a Sanskrit term which means circle, wheel, something round and spinning. There are many chakras in the body, but the major ones form an energy circuit along the spinal column in the region of the five major nerve plexuses. These chakras are mediatory, receiving energy from the higher levels and transmitting it throughout mind and body.

Due to their physical proximity and corresponding functions, the main chakras are often identified with the nerve plexuses or even the glands, but in fact they are neither. The chakras function at a much subtler rate of vibration although it is claimed that they have been located with the aid of acutely sensitive scientific equipment.[1] The chakras at the lowest level of the energy circuit vibrate more slowly in comparison to higher chakras in the throat and head. The rate of vibration in each chakra in turn affects the functioning of the glands and organs to which it is connected, thus influencing the entire body structure as well as the metabolism.

Five, six or seven chakras?
In the human body there are seven main chakras located along the vertebral column and in the head. Of course,

many minor chakras are placed throughout the whole body, and they even exist in the animal, vegetable, and mineral kingdoms. Above the highest chakra related to human evolution, there are also chakras which belong to the divine realm.

All these chakras function at varying vibrational frequencies, and are therefore perceived as vortices of light, which vary in colour depending on their rate of vibration. The rishis who perceived these chakras in deep meditation saw that they resembled lotus flowers of different shades with different numbers of petals. Therefore, in the yogic texts they described them as the lotuses of the body.

The lowest chakra is called mooladhara, then moving up the spine are swadhisthana, manipura, anahata, vishuddhi and ajna. Further up we come to sahasrara. Mooladhara is the equivalent of sahasrara in the animal kingdom. It is from mooladhara that man's primal energy can be transformed into a spiritual force, and it is from there that ida, pingala and sushumna originate. At the end of the circuit they merge again in ajna and proceed as one to sahasrara at the crown of the head.

Sahasrara is totally free from the influences of ida and pingala and, therefore, it is not always considered to be a chakra. Many yogic scriptures only talk about five chakras along the vertebral column, others include ajna, but few include sahasrara. Mooladhara to vishuddhi belong to the range of the five basic elements of creation. Ajna is concerned with mind and intuition alone. In the lower centres, matter is denser and awareness is dimmer, while in the higher centres awareness predominates and matter becomes increasingly more subtle up to sahasrara, which is pure awareness devoid of matter.

Activating the chakras

A chakra can be consciously activated either by directing prana to the centre or by concentrating on its location and form. However, both methods produce the same result because, when you direct pranic energy to a chakra, you become aware of its location, so mental visualization and concentration are also taking place. When you concentrate on the chakra or a symbol which stimulates it, prana also moves to that centre. So the two systems are basically one.

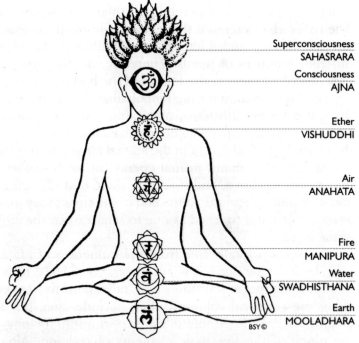

Superconsciousness
SAHASRARA
Consciousness
AJNA
Ether
VISHUDDHI
Air
ANAHATA
Fire
MANIPURA
Water
SWADHISTHANA
Earth
MOOLADHARA

Position of the chakras and their related tattwas

However, it is very important to note that awakening of the chakras and awakening of kundalini are different processes. The chakras should be purified before the awakening of kundalini, because they are usually either blocked or operating at a very low vibration. Therefore, first they have to be purified, then activated and attuned to a higher frequency, so that kundalini can pass through without causing any harm or disturbance.

In swara yoga the practice of concentration on the tattwas or elements is utilized to activate the chakras. By analyzing the breath, one finds out which tattwa is active. This means that prana is operating at the level of the corresponding chakra. Thus, by understanding the elements and faculties of each chakra, the signs and indications of awakening can be recognized by the nature of the breath.

DESCRIPTION OF THE CHAKRAS

Mooladhara

The lowest energy centre, mooladhara, is at the base of the spine in the region of the coccygeal plexus. *Mool* means root and *adhara* place. All the basic animal urges arise from this centre and it is where human evolution begins. Mooladhara influences the excretory and reproductive organs and glands. It is connected to the nasal cavity and sense of smell and can therefore be stimulated from the nose tip, as in nasikagra drishti.

Symbolically, mooladhara is represented by a four-petalled red lotus. Inside is a yellow square surrounded by a circle, which represents the earth element. All the physical and subtle qualities of the earth element manifest from the level of mooladhara. The swara yogi meditates on a yantra of the earth element to awaken the inherent potential of mooladhara.

Swadhisthana

Two fingers above mooladhara in the sacral plexus lies swadhisthana. *Swa* means self, *sthana* means place. When consciousness and energy operate in swadhisthana, awareness of self and ego is aroused. Swadhisthana is closely linked to mooladhara and also influences the reproductive organs and glands. The word *swad* refers to taste and tasting is the specific sensorial faculty associated with swadhisthana. The ability to taste is dependent on the sense of smell and in the same way swadhisthana is dependent on mooladhara.

Swadhisthana is symbolized by a six-petalled vermilion lotus. There is a circle inside and at the bottom a crescent moon. The crescent moon represents the inherent water element. Over the crescent moon is the deep, dark ocean, above which is the moonlit night. All these represent the subconscious mind. To arouse the faculties of swadhisthana, the swara yogi practices trataka on the yantra of the water element, but gazing at the crescent moon at night is also effective.

Manipura

Behind the navel in the solar plexus is manipura chakra. *Mani* means jewel, *puri* means city. Manipura is the city of jewels. At this point the nadis congregate, radiating immense light, and the yogic texts describe it as shining like a lustrous jewel. Manipura contains the fire element, which thus explains the expression 'digestive fire'.

Manipura is concerned with digestion and absorption of food and prana. It is referred to as the midpoint between earth and heaven because in the lower centres the awareness is oriented towards gross experience, but when it passes through manipura, higher ideals develop. Manipura is the midpoint between the physical body and the point where the yogic texts say that prana and apana have to be united. We can say manipura is the turning point from gross to subtle. It is symbolized by a bright yellow lotus of ten petals in which there is an inverted triangle and blazing red fire. The inner yantra represents the inherent fire element, and in the practice of swara yoga you concentrate on this inner yantra.

Manipura is of great importance to the swara yogi for two reasons. One, because it is the centre where prana is stored, and two, because the goddess Lakshmi resides there. The *Shiva Swarodaya* says that Lakshmi blesses and protects the practitioner of swara yoga. She is the creative power of Lord Vishnu, the cosmic preserver, and the deity of wealth, prosperity and good fortune. The concept of Lakshmi is symbolic of the effects of activating manipura and stimulating the prana and consciousness to this level of vibration.

Anahata

The cardiac plexus is the next important centre, which is known as anahata chakra. *Ana* means no, *ahata* means struck. In the heart centre is the unstruck vibration of the eternal nada. It is where the pulse of the universe and pulse of human existence can be experienced. The great tantric guru Gorakhnath said that by constant awareness of each breath, occurring 21,600 times day and night, you can experience the sound produced in the heart centre. Anahata is described as the residing place of the jivatma or individual soul. Thus, perceiving the prana in anahata means coming closer to your inner being.

Anahata is symbolized by a pale blue lotus with twelve petals. Inside are two interlaced triangles, one pointing up, the other down. This yantra represents the air element. The swara yogi performs trataka on the yantra of the air element to realize the pranic potential in anahata and activate it.

Vishuddhi

In the cervical plexus is vishuddhi. *Vi* signifies something great and beyond comparison. *Shuddhi* means purifier. Vishuddhi prevents toxins from circulating through the system. It has a direct influence on the throat, tonsils, vocal cords, thyroid and parathyroid glands. The yogic texts talk about a fluid which falls from a higher chakra and is retained in vishuddhi, where it becomes nectarine, generating vitality and longevity. But when this amrit falls further to manipura, it is burnt, causing eventual disease, old age and death.

Vishuddhi appears as a smoky violet lotus with sixteen petals. In the centre is a white bindu, like the full moon, representing the qualities of vishuddhi and the ether element. It is also symbolic of the purer state of consciousness and prana operating at the high vibrational level of vishuddhi when it is activated. Vishuddhi is known as the 'great gate of liberation' and in swara yoga trataka is practised on the yantra of the ether element to awaken its potential and open the gate.

Ajna

Ajna chakra is very important in tantra and swara yoga. It is located at the top of the spinal column, in the region of the medulla oblongata. This centre is associated with the pineal gland and is known as the guru or command centre, because from ajna, intuition is transmitted to the lower centres and mind. Therefore, ajna is also known as the third eye, or the eye of intuition, the medium between the highest consciousness or guru and the ego or jivatma; between the higher brain faculties and instinctive brain functions.

Ida and pingala merge with sushumna at ajna. Thus it is said that duality ceases at ajna, and so it has been called *mukta triveni*. In the Hindu tradition the merging of ida, pingala and sushumna at ajna is related to the confluence of the three holy rivers, Ganga, Yamuna and Saraswati. Ida and pingala represent the terrestrial rivers, Ganga and Yamuna. Sushumna lying deep within the spinal cord represents the subterranean Saraswati. These three rivers merge at Prayag in northern India just as the three nadis merge at ajna. The place where they converge is a very powerful energy centre, which awakens the higher creative force in man.

The role of ajna is associated with the functions of the pineal gland. The pineal gland is connected to the pituitary gland, which produces a hormone that sets the whole endocrine system into operation and, in particular, controls growth and the activity of the sex glands. When the pineal gland functions, it acts like a lock on the pituitary gland. In most people certain parts of the pineal gland begin to degenerate after the age of eight. Then the pituitary gland comes into full play and the worldly personality develops. As long as the pineal gland remains intact however, certain functions within the pituitary gland are controlled.

The pineal is the guru, the pituitary gland the disciple. This is the proper relationship between the two glands.

66

When the relationship is reversed, then you have all types of emotional, mental, psychic and physical problems. In swara yoga, it is well known that this can be rectified by balancing ida and pingala at ajna. Furthermore, the pineal gland is affected by the light/dark cycles. Likewise, the swara and ida/pingala operate in accordance with these cycles, but if they are out of sequence, it indicates that something is disturbed in the energy circuit between mooladhara and ajna.

The pineal gland enables the extrasensory perceptions like clairvoyance, clairaudience, telepathy, etc. to function. In swara yoga it is essential that these subtler faculties are developed, and a powerful method for stimulating them is trataka. The practice of trataka on the tattwa yantras and on your shadow (chhayopasana) stimulate ajna, though ajna is not specifically influenced by the individual tattwas because it is above the range of these elements. In fact, ajna is described as the seat of the subtlest tattwas, *mahat* or pure consciousness and *prakriti*, the cosmic creative power. In the practice of swara yoga a subtle state of mind is needed to understand the meaning and influence of the individual tattwas. Therefore, it is essential to develop ajna's full capacity.

Sahasrara

Sahasrara is different from the other chakras in constitution and effect. When the kundalini shakti reaches this level, it does not belong to the realm of the animal or human awareness, it is purely divine. Sahasrara is located at the very top of the head and its functions are associated with the pituitary gland. It is the thousand-petalled lotus leading into eternal, infinite, supreme existence. It is the seat of pure consciousness. Mooladhara is the abode of kundalini shakti, and when it rises to sahasrara, where energy and consciousness remain together, illumination dawns. Then, under the influence of ajna, the force created from the meeting of these two is redirected down so that one experiences heaven on earth. Thus the yogi fulfils the meaning of yoga and the purpose of swara yoga is attained.

13

The Pancha Tattwas

The philosophy of tantra and swara yoga explains how the whole universe is the composition of five *maha bhutas* or tattwas. These are the elements of *akasha* (ether), *vayu* (air), *agni* (fire), *apas* (water) and *prithvi* (earth). Ever since the time of ancient civilizations, man has always considered that the world is made up of the four fundamental elements of earth, water, fire and air. These elements represent particular frequencies and states of prana and consciousness.

The *Mandukyopanishad*, *Prashnopanishad* and *Shiva Swarodaya* explain that the five elements or pancha tattwas evolved from mind, mind from prana and prana from super-consciousness. As the human body itself is made up of the same cosmic elements, the properties of these elements are inherent throughout the body right down to the tiniest cell and atom. Their influence is so subtle and precise that they affect the whole pattern of life. Just as the blueprint of all your physical and mental characteristics is contained within the DNA molecule, the combination and proportion of the tattwas also determine the whole structure of your being.

Each tattwa has a particular pranic frequency and affects the mechanisms of the body and flow of prana. Therefore, tattwa sadhana is a practice used in swara yoga to study the flow of the breath in order to recognize the predominant tattwa. These tattwas are indicative of psychophysiological states and cause the breath to flow in different directions on exhalation. If you know which tattwa is active, you can judge your physical, mental and emotional state and gauge it according to whatever task you are about to undertake. But more than this, the practice increases our mundane awareness and experience so that a deeper understanding grows of who and what we are.

Nature of the tattwas

Tattwa is a particular vibration of prana from which specific sound frequencies, *mantra*, and colour or *varna* are created. Prana is pure light, and just as white light contains all the various colours of the spectrum, in the same way, prana can be broken down into the individual tattwas. Scientists have shown that light particles move in particular patterns to create the different rays of light such as infrared, ultra violet or even a laser beam. In much the same way, prana vibrates throughout the body at different frequencies at the speed of red light, blue light, yellow light, etc. These colours and vibrations, when registered as sound, indicate the various tattwas.

The first tattwa which manifested was akasha or ether, so-called because of its subtle, all-pervading and motionless nature. From ether came vayu or air, which is prana in a subtle state, but there is movement, something like the nature of the wind. From vayu, agni (fire) evolved, where prana became hot like fire. As it cooled it became apas (water) and could flow like a stream of water. When it settled, it became immovable, like a rock, prithvi or the earth. In this way the nature of the tattwas indicates the influence and effect of prana when it operates at these particular frequencies.

In the body there are different levels of energy and different pranic movements. The prana is not just moving at random; it follows certain laws. The nadis channel prana into the various chakras situated along the spinal column and the frequencies of these centres increase in vibration

69

from mooladhara up. In yoga we say that the earth tattwa is the lowest and akasha the highest vibration of the individual elements. But it must be remembered here that the tattwas are not physical and chemical elements. They refer to a particular level of energy, sound frequency and light emanation.

In the same way that the chakras have corresponding sensory organs, so each tattwa manifests as an inherent quality of those organs. We know the direct connection between the nose, the sense of smell and mooladhara. Likewise the other tattwas correspond to specific sensory organs. Chapter 2 of the *Prapanchasara Tantra* explains that "akasha is in the ears, vayu in the skin, agni in the eyes, apas in the tongue and prithvi in the nostrils". This indicates the particular centre to which the organs and tattwas are connected and it also gives another clue into the nature of each tattwa.

The quality of earth is smell, water is taste, fire sight, air touch and ether sound. Smell is a primitive brain function and similarly earth is the grossest element. Each tattwa becomes subtler in effect and nature until you enter the realm of consciousness. In swara yoga you develop awareness of the effects of specific tattwas on the functions of the body and thereby come to know how you are affected by different pranic vibrations.

Properties of the tattwas
The tattwas can be recognized in gross, subtle, individual and cosmic manifestations. These tattwas interact with each other and due to this, as the *Shiva Swarodaya* explains, all changes in the universe are effected. The particular characteristics of the tattwas are listed in the following chart (overleaf).

Recognizing the tattwas
In swara yoga the active tattwa can be recognized by the specific length and direction of breath. If you concentrate on

70

Properties of the Tattwas

Element	Earth	Water	Fire	Air	Ether
Nature	heavy	cool	hot	erratic	mixed
Quality	weight, cohesion	fluidity, contraction	heat, expansion	motion, movement	diffused, space giving
Colour	yellow	white	red	blue/grey	blackish with multi-coloured points of light, translucent
Shape	quadrangular	crescent moon	triangular	hexagonal	bindu/dot
Chakra	mooladhara	swadhisthana	manipura	anahata	vishuddhi
Mantra	lam (लं)	vam (वं)	ram (रं)	yam (यं)	ham (हं)
Tanmatra	smell	taste	sight	touch	sound
Function in body	skin, blood vessels, bone construction	all fluids of the body	appetite, thirst, sleep	expansion, contraction of muscles	emotions passions
Location in body	thighs	feet	shoulder region	navel region	forehead
State of mind	ahamkara (ego)	buddhi (discrimination)	manasa (thought, counter-thought)	chitta (psychic content)	pragya (intuition)
Kosha	annamaya	pranamaya	manomaya	vigyanamaya	anandamaya
Prana Vayu	apana	prana	samana	udana	vyana
Planet	mercury	moon and venus	sun and mars	saturn and neptune	jupiter
Direction	east	west	south	north	middle and above

the particular manner in which the breath is flowing in and out, you can know the level at which your prana is operating, your state of mind and what you are capable of achieving at that time.

To become familiar with each tattwa requires intense concentration and sensitivity of mind because as the *Shiva Swarodaya* states, "The tattwas are hidden at a very subtle level of existence." Just as a scientist can only see the molecules comprising matter by looking through a micro- scope, in the same way, swara yoga explains that the tattwas which manifest in various forms can only be perceived by meditating upon the forms of the tattwas. If you recognize the tattwas, you know the nature of your being and of cosmic events.

The flow of prana within the body is affected to various degrees by the external environment and the energy flow in other people. You know what happens when you put two opposite poles of a magnet together, or place the same poles end to end, or put many magnets together side by side, and then bring a metallic object within close range. The result of the interaction depends on the magnetic properties of the interacting objects and the strength of their magnetism.

Similarly, by knowing the active pranic flow or tattwa in the body, you can estimate what is going to happen when you are in particular situations because the magnet- like properties of the tattwas depend on the external environment. It is like seeing a shadow; you know it is created by an object, or when there is smoke, you know there is fire or when it rains, there must be clouds. Similarly, through swara yoga you can know the outcome of events in the past, present or future through the interaction of the pranas and tattwas.

Astrology and swara

The *Shiva Swarodaya* tells how the breath relates to planetary, solar and lunar movements, and it also has some connection with astrology. The *Shiva Swarodaya* also states that astrology without the science of swara is useless. Astrology discusses the influence of four fundamental elements which affect a person's life and character. These are the cosmic elements. Swara yoga talks about the same elements, but says they manifest in the body and can be detected by analyzing the body processes and breath. In astrology the elements represent particular levels of vibration and influence at the cosmic level. In swara yoga these elements and vibrations are seen to be present within the individual structure. So we do not have to look into the universe because the macrocosm is mirrored in the microcosm.

Swara yoga and astrology are like the two ends of the same stick. In India, the calculations of the Hindu astrological system are so precise that the exact time of the swara can be predicted. In the Hindu system there are nine main periods in the day over which a planet presides, and these periods are divided and subdivided until you reach the exact second of the swara, the moment of inhalation and exhalation. Astrology is based on the planets and swara yoga on the breath. By becoming aware of the swara and tattwas, we also become aware of those cosmic influences which affect our health and destiny, and can therefore make better use of good opportunities and find ways to ameliorate our malefic influences. Thus the yogic texts say that regulation of the breath and pranayama help to destroy the bonds of worldly existence.

Some scientists have observed certain relationships between cosmic events and individual experiences, social and cultural events. We can assume that the brain and CNS are receptive to the force fields of planetary and stellar radiations and movements, and some scientists are investigating this interaction.[1] Today man is looking into the sky to understand himself better, but to the swara yogi there is no difference between cosmic and atomic events. It is not necessary to understand astrophysics, because everyone has the capacity to close their eyes, look into the dark space of their consciousness and experience the worlds within.

73

Making predictions

Through recognizing the active element in the breath, you can come to know the future. There are a number of astrologers in India who can usually make reliable offhand predictions. For example, if a student asks, "Sir, will I pass or fail?" he will first check the day and then feel his breath. If it is positive, he will say, "Yes," and if it is negative, "No." This is how some people have misused the science, but this is not its purpose. It is not the science which is at fault but the person's motives. So we should be careful of such people and remember the true purpose of this science.

Practices According
to the Swara Shastras

14

Prana Sadhana

To have *atma anubhuti*, experience of the universal spirit, is the destiny of man. In order to have that experience, the part of the mind which functions and perceives the external world through the senses has to be jumped over. The mind has to become so concentrated and one-pointed that it is completely still without the minutest fluctuation or wavering. The moment the mind stops, the breath too is suspended. The consciousness and prana can then slip out of the individual range of experience.

It is a difficult process because one is faced with many obstacles which lure the mind away from its point of focus. The obstacles have to be overcome if progress is to be made in this very life. But is it possible for everybody to experience and understand their own atma – the true Self? Yoga and tantra say yes. Even the *Bhagavad Gita* gives assurance that everybody has the right to realize the highest experience of life. But the problem is that we do not make enough effort. To do any practice takes time, and we have to fight with the mind. Sometimes we are inspired for a month or two and concentration becomes very keen, but again inspiration dies and the battery becomes flat. Then other obstacles come like disease, laziness, fulfilment of worldly desires and samskaras, etc.

The yoga shastras say that when the pranas are disturbed, the mind is also disturbed. Therefore, yoga devised two ways to overcome this. The first states that if the pranas are controlled, the mind can also be controlled because the two are interrelated and interdependent. This path involves hatha and swara yoga. The other path says that when the mind becomes disturbed, the pranas are disturbed, and if the mind is controlled, the pranas also come under control. That is the path of raja and jnana yoga.

Controlling the prana is like controlling an elephant. If you can do it, you are its master. But to control the mind is like trying to control the air. Therefore, people today find it much easier and more tangible to deal with the prana, provided, of course, that they have a guru.

Raja yoga sets out eight steps: yama, niyama, asana, pranayama, pratyahara, dharana, dhyana and samadhi. The ancient hatha yoga texts rearranged these into a suitable order for the people of Kali yuga, starting with the shatkarmas – neti, dhauti, basti, kapalbhati, trataka and nauli. Later texts such as *Hatha Yoga Pradipika* added asana and pranayama. The order of yama/niyama coming first had to be changed, because people found it difficult to meditate and tackle the problem of higher experience when the mundane problems were overpowering them. Those who can practise have to deal with the problems of the world and they suffer because of infirmity of will. So now the practice of the shatkarmas comes first. Control the prana and the mind will become quiet. You will have a clear mind to analyze the pranic movements and practise yoga.

The shatkarmas are done to purify the physical body, as well as the nadis and chakras. They strengthen and stimulate the whole system. After practising hatha yoga, you will experience lightness of body and clarity of mind. At the same time, you will spontaneously notice the subtle flow of prana, ida/pingala and perhaps even sushumna.

In the *Shiva Swarodaya* the practices of moola bandha and maha bandha are also mentioned. Practice of the three bandhas: jalandhara bandha, uddiyana bandha and moola bandha, in combination with breath retention (kumbhaka), and shambhavi mudra, helps to increase the capacity of the pranic force. Therefore, hatha yoga and raja yoga are necessary for swara yoga. In fact, they are not separate compartments, they are all complementary. The hatha yoga shatkarmas aid pranayama, pranayama aids raja yoga, and swara yoga gives deeper insight into both systems.

Balancing ida and pingala

The famous guru Gorakhnath, the greatest exponent of hatha yoga, used to tell his disciples that when they practised hatha yoga, they were not doing mere exercise. They were not just purifying the physical body. They were trying to bring about a balance between the two forces in the body, known as the sun and moon. In the word hatha, *ha* represents the sun, and *tha*, the moon. So, ha and tha represent pingala and ida, the solar and lunar forces.

Hatha yoga brings a balance between the alternating activities of the two nadis. It ensures that they operate in rhythm with the movements of the external sun and moon. Secondly, it increases the capacity of all the nadis, vayus and chakras. By incorporating swara yoga, a total balance in the nadis and awakening of sushumna can take place.

Prerequisites

Before you begin the advanced swara practices, the whole body system should be clean and functioning rhythmically so that your results may be accurate. The practices are easier and more effective when there are no digestive, respiratory or nasal defects. Therefore, you should at least be practising asana, pranayama and one or two of the shatkarmas such as neti and kunjal.

Swara yoga is comparable to kriya or kundalini yoga in its demands on your capacity and actual knowledge of yoga. Of course, there are simple and easy practices which anyone can utilize any time of the day or night, but the core of swara yoga requires that you are comfortable in your meditative posture and proficient in pranayama, mudra, bandha, trataka, visualization and japa. The application of the major practices are for advanced students and sadhakas.

Therefore, if you are serious about the practice and not just trying it out, you will also have to regulate your lifestyle. The swara shastras state that the diet should be *mitahara*, which means balanced, nutritious and pure. The practitioner should neither eat too much nor too little, so that the body and mind remain steady and alert. Secondly, it is beneficial to avoid oversleeping: six to seven hours is quite sufficient. Get up early and sleep early. When you sleep late the mind and body become dull. Thirdly, it is necessary to have a steady and unfluctuating state of mind and to practise regularly. There is no point in stopping and starting the practices because you will not get anywhere. Of course, simple awareness of the swara and how to act during the flow of ida, pingala and sushumna can be done, but those who want to gain steadiness of mind will have to be regular.

In fact, steadiness of mind means that whatever you gain from the practices mentally, physically or psychically should be utilized for spiritual evolution. If you gain greater mental and psychic capacity than your business associates or your next door neighbour, save it for your inner enlightenment rather than wasting it on selfish purposes that only better your material position.

Swara yoga can open a whole new vista of life to the practitioner. However, it is essential to remind yourself that the science was not designed to bestow *siddhis* or psychic powers. Though such side effects can manifest, keep in mind that the ultimate goal for which you are striving is to heighten your consciousness beyond mundane experiences.

15

Explanation of the Practices

If you can understand the nature of the breath, you can definitely gain greater insight into the body and mind. If you can control the swara, you can control the activities of the brain and nervous system. This is based on the fact that when the left nostril flows, there is activity in the right brain hemisphere, and when the right nostril flows, the left hemisphere is active. This influences the functioning of the entire system.

Therefore, it is important that the alternating cycles of ida and pingala are systematic. Every three days the nadis change their sequence at the time of sunrise. During the bright fortnight when the moon is waxing (increasing) and the dark fortnight when it is waning (decreasing), the moment the sun rises there is a predetermined order of the swara. If your swara does not follow the correct sequence, there is a defect in your system.

The breath flowing in the right or left nostril has to flow in the systematic order according to the movements of the sun and moon. That is why ida and pingala are referred to as lunar and solar nadis. Ida is cool like the moon, and pingala hot like the sun. Yogis in highly developed meditative states of consciousness report that they experience a difference in temperature between the air that flows through the right and left nostrils. This is an indication of the inner body temperature and functions. It is fluctuating between 'warm' and 'cool'.

Therefore, if both the swaras operate together, there is perfect balance in every respect. But this has to be developed.

What do the swara yogis do? They make their surya swara flow by night and chandra swara by day. This brings a balance between the external forces and internal functions. They sit in a particular asana, *padadhirasana*, which is specially designed for changing the swara. First they have to observe whether the correct swara is flowing at the right time. Then it may have to be changed accordingly. For this purpose they use a special stick called a *yoga danda*, which rests under the arm, to change the flow of the swara.

Separation and union

The different flows of shakti in the body create different vibrational patterns. Those vibrations are the tattwas of akasha, vayu, agni, apas and prithvi. This does not mean the sky above our heads, the air we breathe, the fire that burns us, the water we drink, the earth of minerals and plants. The tattwas are symbolic of the various types of energy vibration and their function and effect.

These vibrations can only be perceived by the subtle mind. When you close your eyes, you see different colours in *chidakasha*, the canvas of your mind; sometimes yellow, sometimes blue, white, red or grey. As the level of prana in the body alters, we say the tattwa is changing. Each tattwa has a specific colour or *varna*. These tattwas keep on flowing like electrons. When you can perceive this flow, spiritual experience begins. These spiritual experiences belong to all the koshas.

The deeper you go, the greater the experiences become. And what are these experiences? These are experiences of the invisible bodies; the *sukshma sharira* (subtle body) and *karana sharira* (causal body). So when we use the word 'body', let us understand the *loka* or plane of existence to which it relates.

We do not only exist on the conscious plane, which we know through the senses. According to the shastras, there are seven planes of existence. As consciousness becomes free from matter and vibrates at a higher frequency, we ascend from bhuh loka to bhuvah loka, svah loka, mahah loka, janah loka, tapah loka and satya loka. These lokas represent the state of our existence as we progress into the more subtle realms. Progress depends on the freedom and liberation of the mind from matter. When mind and matter are separated, then there is a release of energy.

In one of his poems Kabir has said, "Within the framework of this body, there is a great wonder; there is a couple, male and female." This directly alludes to the idea of ida and pingala. He also said, "Those who are able to unite this couple can separate them." These are the two processes which take place in yoga and tantra side by side. First, there is union between ida and pingala, between meditator and the object of meditation, prana and mind. The moment it takes place, matter and energy are separated.

That is the purpose of yoga, the separation of energy from matter. Union is not the purpose of yoga, it is the means. Whom do you unite? You are uniting yourself with the object of meditation, uniting the meditator and object of meditation, *upasaka* and *upasya*. The moment this union takes place, meditation occurs. That is what we call separation of matter and energy. *Padartha*, or the object, and the inherent shakti are separated. This separation of energy from matter is awakening of kundalini.

When awakening of kundalini takes place, whether you are illiterate or learned, or have no *bhakti* (devotion) at all, you will at once start having experiences. These experiences lead from one state to another, as the energy rises from the lower centres, mooladhara and swadhisthana, to the higher centres, manipura, anahata, vishuddhi, ajna and sahasrara. The six chakras, from mooladhara to ajna plus sahasrara, represent the seven lokas or planes of our progressive consciousness.

The path to higher experience
In order to release shakti and inner experiences, there is not one but thousands of ways. First, you will have to approach a

suitable guru and read the yogic texts. You have to know the dimensions and structure of your whole being.

Swara yoga is just one of the ways to experience the more subtle aspect of your being. It is a process of self-analysis to be incorporated into your daily life, and should be utilized with other spiritual practices in order to enhance, understand and control the mundane experiences.

This is not a path of blind faith. Nor is it a path for the superstitious. It is a path for those who are seekers, and seekers can never be blind followers. They search, analyze, and come to their own realizations, ultimately to find the truth of existence.

16

Recognizing the Swara

We start the practice of swara yoga by learning how to recognize which nadi and swara is functioning. When the flow of air is coming from the left nostril only, ida is active, and this is known as the *vama* or left swara. When the right nostril is open, pingala is active, and it is called *dakshina* or right swara. Recognizing the active swara is a simple process; exhale into the palm of the hand and you will feel a stronger current flow from the open nostril.

If you are still unsure after testing in this way, then close one nostril and breathe out through the other. Listen for a difference in the pitch of right and left exhalation. The deeper sound indicates the open nostril, the higher pitch indicates the closed. Sometimes both nostrils flow equally and you cannot differentiate whether the right or left is predominant. This is the flow of sushumna or *shoonya swara*.

Length of the prana
When you are examining which nostril is active, at different times during the day you will notice that the length of the breath alters. Sometimes it is longer or shorter. According to the swara shastras, the aim of the practice is to reduce the length of the exhaled breath so that more prana is retained in the body.

The swara shastras give the length of the natural expiration during particular activities. The distance is given

85

in the measurement of an *angula* or one finger's breath. Of course, measurements are given for the normal healthy person but other factors of age, weight, height, etc. should also be taken into consideration.

- The natural length is 7–12 angulas.
- During states of emotion and excitation 12–36 angulas.
- While singing 16 angulas.
- Vomiting 18 angulas.
- Eating 20 angulas.
- Walking 24 angulas.
- Sleeping 30 angulas.
- Exercise and copulation 36 angulas.
- Strenuous physical exertion 36–100 angulas.

During the day spontaneous emphasis is on inhalation. People with weak constitutions project the expiration to a longer distance. If the breath extends further than 8 inches while lying flat, excess energy is being lost.

Reducing the length of the swara

The *Shiva Swarodaya* claims that those who can expire with the least possible projection of exhalation retain their vital energy and thus develop *siddhis* or perfection of pranic and mental abilities.

- Continuous exhalation which does not exceed the length of one angula, brings about a state of detachment, where you can work without calculating your gain, free from desire (*nishkam*). It will help you become honest and straightforward (*nishkapat*), so that you can remain impartial (*nishpaksha*) and unbiased in any situation.
- Expiration which does not exceed two angulas will keep you happy and content in any situation. You will attain anandam.
- Breath of three angulas awakens poetic abilities.
- Exhalation of four angulas gives *vach siddhi* (i.e. whatever you say comes to pass).
- Expiration of five angulas develops foresight so you can perceive the outcome of an event before it eventuates.

Pranayama

The *Shiva Swarodaya* recommends the practice of pranayama to help develop, regulate and control the length of the prana. That is what the word *pranayama* means, 'length of prana'. *Ayama* is length or extension. Pranayama is usually defined as control of the breath, because people divide the word into *prana* and *yama* (control). However, the real aim of pranayama is to extend the prana into previously dormant areas of the body, brain and personality so as to awaken various inherent faculties and sensitize perception. This is achieved through regulation of the breath, which brings about regulation and storage of prana.

One of the main objects of practising pranayama with breath retention is to activate sushumna, shoonya swara. Therefore, all the pranayamas are helpful, but swara yoga specifies the use of nadi shodhana for gaining awareness and control over the swara. Nadi shodhana is the method of alternate nostril breathing. The *Shiva Swarodaya* says one should first breathe in through the lunar swara and then out through the solar swara, and repeat the process from the solar swara. Inhalation and exhalation have to be controlled in definite proportions, and later breath retention is included.

Inhalation, exhalation and retention all have a specific significance and effect. Inhalation or *pooraka* draws vitality into the body. It is symbolic of creation. Exhalation or *rechaka* eliminates physical impurities and even those at a subtler level. The *Shiva Swarodaya* says it "destroys bad karma" or negative mental impressions. It represents destruction or transformation. *Kumbhaka* or retention generates greater vital capacity. By perfecting these three aspects of the breath, conscious control is gained and one can "exist as long as the moon and stars".

Balancing the breath

The practice of nadi shodhana is considered essential for the practice of swara yoga because it establishes consistency in the breath. Normally, inspiration and expiration come and go in unequal proportions. Either inspiration is not full and expiration very long or vice versa. This shows there is an imbalance of prana in the nadis. Rhythmic breathing in and out has to be established for accurate practice of swara yoga.

The nature of the breath becomes absolutely and comprehensively correct through the practice of nadi shodhana. It is not sufficient to breathe in the usual way. The breath has to become subtle. When the breath is gross, you can feel it at a distance beyond two fingers. The shorter the distance, the more subtle the breath. Exhalation should be in such a way that it does not extend more that two fingers length, but it must still be complete. During pranayama if you are not accustomed to subtle breathing, you will retain the breath and then exhale or inhale too forcefully. This has to be kept in mind during natural breathing as well as pranayama practice.

The speed of inhalation and exhalation is the next important point. It should be consistent. For example, when you are tired, inhalation is deep and slow, exhalation is quick. When you are not tired, you may inhale quickly and exhale slowly and deeply. This is inconsistency in the breathing and creates uneven waves of physical and mental energy which disturb the mind and body. Therefore, consistency is most essential.

Besides consistency, there must be uniformity in the breath. Many people breathe in and out with a slight jerk. The breath should be smooth and uniform without any stopping or jerking. If you study the way people breathe, you will see that it is rarely perfectly uniform for any length of time. In pranayama, after internal or external retention, it is particularly noticeable. During just one exhalation there may be up to ten different speeds until uniformity is established. So, whether you are practising pranayama or just breathing, make it a habit to breathe gently with consistency and uniformity and make the breath subtle.

17

Timing the Swara

As we have already said, ida, pingala and sushumna do not flow at random but at specific times in synchronization with the solar/lunar rhythms. According to the *Shiva Swarodaya*, the active nadi flows for two and a half *ghati*, which is equivalent to 60 minutes. Thereafter, sushumna functions for 1–4 minutes and then the other nadi begins to operate.

Neurologists have found the same sequence in brain hemisphere activity. One hemisphere remains active for 60–90 minutes.[1] When that cycle is complete, there is a transfer of energy to the other hemisphere through a thin sheet of membrane called the corpus callosum, over a period of 1–4 minutes. Science has also found that the brain hemispheres control breathing in the right and left nostrils. The active hemisphere stimulates the connected nostril, therefore, there is always one nostril active while the other remains partially blocked.[2]

To know the exact time when ida/pingala become active, you will need to be acquainted with the moon phases. During the first 14 days (*tithis*)* of the lunar cycle (which extends

---

Tithi is the date of the lunar month, it is not the date of the solar month. You will notice that 30 tithis are listed in the lunar month, and it must be remembered that the time of the lunar tithi varies in comparison to the solar day. In 28 solar days there are 30 lunar tithis. It is an involved system, and a lunar calendar is required to tell the lunar tithi.

from the new moon to the full moon), the moon waxes and becomes fuller. This is called *shukla paksha* or bright fortnight: shukla means white, and paksha means fortnight. On the 15th tithi the moon is full; this is called *poornima*. During the next 14 tithis of the cycle (i.e. between the full moon and the new moon) the moon wanes and becomes darker. This is known as the *krishna paksha*, krishna meaning black. On the 15th tithi, called *amavasya*, there is no moon.

In the swara cycle surya nadi (pingala) becomes active at sunrise during krishna paksha on tithis 1-3, 7-9, 13-15. Thereafter, ida and pingala function alternately in 60-90 minute cycles throughout the day until at sunset, chandra nadi (ida) begins to function on the specified days. On tithis 4-6, 10-12 of krishna paksha, the chandra nadi flows at sunrise and surya nadi at sunset. During shukla paksha we see the reverse. At sunrise of the first 3 tithis, chandra nadi flows, etc.

In the process of applying and validating the ancient texts, people coming from all religions and cultures have undertaken swara yoga sadhana. In 90% of cases, this system was observed to be operating.

In timing the swara, the time of sunrise is an important consideration. In summer the sun rises earlier than in winter, and the time is constantly changing throughout the year. The time will also differ according to the exact location and hemisphere of the continent on which you are living. In India the sun rises between 4.45 and 5.15 am in summer, and in winter between 6.15 and 6.45 am. Before the actual sunrise, however, it is already quite bright. This means that the specified nadi flows around the time of sunrise.

Of course, those people who live in the city and are surrounded by tall buildings will not be able to tell the time of sunrise just by looking at the sky. If the sky is covered by pollution, you will have to check with a newspaper even to know where the moon is.

When you first start observing your swara, it is advisable to make a diary of your own swara activities. However, you

Swara Timetable

Day of the moon (tithi)	Bright fortnight (shukla paksha)	Dark fortnight (krishna paksha)
1st/prathama 2nd/dwitiya 3rd/tritiya	chandra swara (ida)	surya swara (pingala)
4th/chaturthi 5th/panchami 6th/shashth	surya swara (pingala)	chandra swara (ida)
7th/saptami 8th/ashtami 9th/naumi	chandra swara (ida)	surya swara (pingala)
10th/dashami 11th/ekadashi 12th/dwadashi	surya swara (pingala)	chandra swara (ida)
13th/trayodashi 14th/chaturdashi 15th/amavasya/ poornima	chandra swara (ida)	surya swara (pingala)

have to keep your diary with you and on an hourly basis, or half-hourly if possible, make a note of which swara is active. This will help you in your practice and simultaneously you will become acquainted with your own rhythm. You may even notice the occurrence of particular events coinciding with specific rhythms. If you have the opportunity, compare with other people's charts.

Biological rhythms
In the 1970s, science coined the word 'chronopsychology' for the 24 hour cycle. Chronopsychologists found that during the 24 hour cycle certain events and one's mental, emotional and physical abilities have a 'best' or 'most likely' time of day. The *Shiva Swarodaya* says the same and further specifies the times when tasks are either *shubha* (auspicious) or *ashubha* (inauspicious). The swara yogi knows that during the influence of either ida or pingala only certain things can be undertaken if you want to be successful.

Scientists have postulated that external forces set the biological clock by stimulating the pineal gland, which is affected by dark/light cycles. These rhythms, which were previously known to the ancient rishis, show that man is actually only rediscovering himself in relation to the cosmos.

Readjusting the swara

If the right or left swara happens to function out of synchronization with the solar/lunar cycles, then any one of the following methods can be used to readjust the cycle. Of course, it is possible that during your analysis of the swara, you may find other convenient methods to alter the flows.

1. Close the active nostril with either your finger or a piece of cotton wool and breathe through the inactive nostril for 5–10 minutes.
2. Inhale through the active nostril and exhale through the inactive nostril.
3. Apply pressure to the armpit on the same side as the active nostril. After some time the opposite nostril will become activated. For this purpose, the yogis have a stick called the yoga danda which they rest in the armpit. Or you can sit in vajrasana and place the left hand in the right armpit, and right hand in the left armpit. This is called padadhirasana. By altering pressure of the hands you can either regulate the flow or change it completely.
4. Lie on the same side as the active swara. In this position you can also use any of the first three methods.
5. The external environment also influences nasal activities. A sudden blast of hot or cold air or wind can change the swara. Washing the body, or just the face, in extremely hot or cold water automatically changes the flow.
6. The type of food consumed will also affect ida/pingala. Foods which heat the body, such as cayenne pepper (chilli powder) and ginger, directly stimulate surya nadi, whereas foods which cool the system, such as yoghurt and bananas, activate chandra nadi.

18

Personal Observations of Swara Activities

As a part of their training, some sannyasins of Bihar School of Yoga, Munger, practised swara sadhana for a period of six months. Each sadhaka closely observed the swara cycles in relation to the effects on the mind, body and circumstances. One disciple practised this sadhana in greater detail, noting the swara on a half-hour to one hour basis. The result of these observations corresponded to the swara yoga teaching, and further conclusions were also derived. Of course, certain factors of lifestyle, diet and climate have to be taken into consideration: rising at 3.30–4.00 am, sleeping at 9.30–10.00 pm, vegetarian diet, fasting, menstrual cycle, and practice of asana, pranayama, japa and meditation.

Conclusions

- The cycles of ida/pingala start as calculated in the *Shiva Swarodaya*.
- Sixty minutes is the shortest duration of a cycle. The periods before dawn and in the afternoon often extend to three hours.[1]
- Comparison of a few people's swara rhythms showed that at sunrise the swaras usually coincided, but as the day progressed the active periods of each nadi began to vary. Possibly this is due to different kinds of work, involvement with different types of people, different metabolism and

biorhythmic cycles. By evening, however, the cycles usually began to synchronize again.

- It was generally found that pingala flows from 10–10.30 am. In the ashram this is the specified time for taking lunch because the digestive power reaches a peak.
- At twelve o'clock midday the flow of sushumna is generally more common. By 12.30 ida often comes into operation and there is a noticeable lull of energy, externally and internally.
- When one swara predominates for more than three consecutive days, some type of mental, physical or emotional crisis arises.
- A constant flow of ida for more than three days coincides with some respiratory problem such as blocked nose, colds or constipation.
- Continual flow of pingala for more than three days coincides with fever or even boils.
- The onset of menstruation is characterized by the constant flow of one nadi, usually sushumna, sometimes ida, rarely pingala. On the second day ida flows to a greater extent and by the third day the swara alternations become more balanced.
- Bowel movements are facilitated by the flow of pingala and the movement occurs more often during the onset of pingala. When ida is flowing the motion is less free, sometimes even causing constipation.
- Weather tends to influence the flow of the nadis. During heavy rains and cold winds, ida begins to flow; during hot winds, pingala can start to flow constantly. Balanced weather patterns coincide with balanced swara cycles.
- Eating a lot of chillies, black pepper, ginger and other hot spices results in the flow of pingala. Banana taken on an empty stomach, milk, curd or cold drinks (especially ice) activate the left nostril. If the nose is slightly blocked, drinking sweet black coffee can open the nasal passage.
- Splashing the face or anus with hot or extremely cold water can change the flow in the nostrils.

- Intense and continual kirtan or japa induces sushumna or ida to flow for a extensive period.
- The practice of basti automatically activates sushumna.
- Different types of work can alter the flow of the swara. The amount of mental involvement also coincides with the preponderant nadi. If physical work is being done and pingala is flowing, there is complete involvement with the work and actions. If ida happens to flow, the mind starts to wander and one thinks of something else. When sushumna flows, there is awareness of both the physical actions and thought process.
- The flow of the particular nadi affects the physical capacities to perform a task. It is more difficult to apply full physical capacity when ida is active.
- Instructing and inspiring people during the flow of pingala coincides with attentiveness and enthusiasm from the listeners. Instructions come across with more dynamism and influence when pingala flows rather than ida. If sushumna flows, it is much more difficult to captivate people.
- Different months are characterized by different swara patterns. During the monthly cycle, one swara usually predominates and particular predicaments coincide with the excessive flow of one swara. In a Tamil text called the *Swara Chintamani*, it is said that pingala should flow predominantly during the months corresponding to the zodiac signs of Aries, Gemini, Leo, Libra, Sagittarius and Aquarius; and ida should predominate in the months of Pisces, Taurus, Cancer, Scorpio and Capricorn; or pingala should flow during the first six months and ida during the last six. "When the swara flows in this manner there are great comforts."
- It should be kept in mind that the months of the Hindu zodiac divisions are based on the lunar calendar, and therefore the zodiac signs occur at slightly different times than the solar calendar of 364 1/4 days. Nevertheless, it was found on this basis that there is a natural tendency

for one swara to predominate during the months of different zodiacs. When it flows against the proper rhythms there are external difficulties, but when the correct swara predominates, circumstances are both smooth and pleasant.

- Charts of the swara cycle were also compared to the individual biorhythm charts. It was found that there were days when the energy level was exactly between the peak and low phases. Such days are called 'caution days' for physical, emotional and intellectual activity. That is, such activity does not usually prosper on those days. Correspondingly, there is a marked tendency for sushumna to flow for extended periods during this time, suggesting that it would be appropriate to do spiritual practice.
- During a physical caution day, if pingala happens to become excessive, fever can result.
- During emotional caution days, if ida predominates, some emotional disturbance can arise, even an outburst or slight mental depression.
- During an intellectual caution day, if ida is prominent, it coincides with excessive mental activity, fantasy or worry.
- If the caution days of the physical, emotional and intellectual cycles are in close proximity and a particular swara is predominating, some sort of disturbance and imbalance occurs and unpleasant situations may arise.
- During peak and low phases of the cycles, the swara is usually balanced for half the day, then one swara starts to predominate. When the low phases of one cycle coincide with those of another, it also affects which swara will be predominant. Therefore, it is very difficult to come to more definite conclusions in relation to biorhythms.

These are the major trends and patterns found over six months of swara sadhana. Yet it should be kept in mind, that to make a complete and thorough study for yourself can take many years of observation. It is also necessary to observe a group of people under various circumstances and living in different parts of the world.

19

Working with the Active Swara

During the flow of ida or pingala, certain actions are considered more appropriate than others. When ida flows it is *shubha*, auspicious or the right time for:
* Drinking water or urinating
* Getting out of bed
* Calm and silent work, especially that which requires mental creativity
* Purchasing jewellery
* Charity and helping others
* Settling disagreements
* Approaching those in senior positions
* Religious practices, ceremonies, marriage, and initiation of any sort
* Mantra sadhana
* Meeting the guru
* A long journey
* Sowing seeds
* Anything to do with medicines and treatment of diseases
* Singing, playing, composing or listening to music
* Women to participate in sexual relations.

During the flow of pingala it is auspicious for:
* Physical activity and hard work
* Eating, drinking alcohol and evacuating the bowels
* Risky and heroic feats, warfare and challenging ventures

- Shatkarma, kunjal kriya, etc.
- Intellectual study, mathematics, etc.
- Agriculture
- Buying and selling, commerce
- Travel
- Opposition, resistance, accusing or sentencing
- Riding on horseback (motor bikes, etc.)
- Men to engage in sexual intercourse or attracting women.

When the swara is flowing through both nostrils and sushumna or the shoonya swara is active, it is better to do work which requires minimum exertion or attention. 'Shoonya' indicates the state of mind aroused when sushumna is stimulated. The mind becomes less involved with the physical world. The shoonya swara is even referred to as the 'evil' or 'wicked' swara or nadi because, if you have any intentions or expectations of material profit and success, your hopes can be ruined at that time. If death is due, then surely it will occur when this swara is predominant for a long time.

As far as the yogic texts are concerned, there are only two types of fruitful action which should be done during the shoonya swara; one is *yoga abhyasa,* or yogic practices, and the other is some type of fearsome or evil action which requires a completely steady and one-pointed mind. Therefore, the *Shiva Swarodaya* advises that actions which lead to attainment of moksha should be done at that time. The text states in unequivocal terms that it is foolishness to undertake physical action or mental work when the shoonya breath is flowing. However, if you sit for meditation, you will not have any difficulty at all.

Checking the swara before acting

When you have understood and observed the flow of your swara and practised working in correspondence to the active nadi, then you can apply other practices so that each daily activity meets with the most possible success. The swara shastras give the following recommendations:

98

- On waking, determine which swara is active. Touch that side of the nostril and face with the corresponding hand.
- Step out of bed with the foot that corresponds to the active swara; make sure to place that foot on the ground first. If pingala is active, walk with the right foot towards the east or north. If ida is active, walk with the left foot towards the west or south. (Perhaps this explains the significance of getting out of bed 'on the wrong side'.)
- Start work during the flow of the lunar swara.
- When the solar swara is functioning and you eat hot, pungent, sour and oily food, it can overheat the system and cause acidity. Therefore, it is advisable to eat such things during the flow of ida. Likewise, it is better to avoid cold food, ice, etc., or food which cools the system like yoghurt, etc., during the flow of the lunar swara.
- If you take a bath in cold water, make sure pingala is active.
- Or if you take a bath in hot water, make sure ida is active.
- The *Swara Chintamani* also advises checking the sequence between bowel movements and urination. Urinating at the time of the left swara, ida, is a healthy sign. If you have planned any venture, it will meet with success. But if the urine comes at intervals, the prana is not functioning optimally, especially if urination is during the right swara. This is an indication of worry or anxiety and troubles. First urine should come, then excreta, then gas. This is a sign of success in any plan. But if all three come together at once, definitely the system is disturbed and there is some pranic imbalance between ida and pingala.
- When commencing a journey, before leaving the house or city start with the foot corresponding to the active nadi and nostril.
- If you wish to approach a person in a friendly manner, especially one with whom you tend to have some conflict, start towards him/her with the same foot as the active nostril. During your interactions with that person keep the inactive side towards him/her.

- While giving orders, face the person from the side of the active swara.
- A woman can attract a man from the side of her flowing lunar swara. Vice versa, a man can attract a woman from the side of his active solar swara.
- When accepting or offering something, use the hand corresponding to the active swara.

Swara – key to health

The state of our body and mind is reflected in the alternation of the swara cycles. If either nadi predominates for too long, it is a sign or warning that one of the branches of the autonomic nervous system is being overstressed and only one of the brain hemispheres is being fully utilized. If ida flows for a long time beyond the normal schedule, this signifies some imbalance in the mind. Or if pingala flows beyond schedule, there is some sort of imbalance in the pranic body. When the physical and mental energies are unbalanced, the personality is only half developed and sickness of some type is inevitable. In order to correct this situation there must be regular alternation of the swara.

The type of sickness which occurs generally indicates which nadi and energy system has been flowing excessively. Many problems resulting from poor digestion such as flatulence, indigestion, diarrhoea, dysentery, cholera and dyspepsia, as well as respiratory disorders and male impotence, are associated with excessive flow of ida. On the other hand, such stress related problems as hypertension, acidity and ulcers arise from the overactivation of pingala.

The *Shiva Swarodaya* advises that for good health the sadhaka and yogi should maximize the flow of ida during the day and the flow of pingala at night. We should keep in mind that the yogi's life is dedicated to sadhana and not household duties. Nevertheless, by adjusting the swara in such a way, the natural tendency of the body to become overheated during the day and overcool at night is counterbalanced with wide-reaching effects.

The overheating and undercooling of the body can be rectified by a correct sleeping position at night. In fact, an investigation carried out in India showed that out of 48 dyspeptic patents two-thirds slept on their right side as opposed to their left. The control group consisted of seven healthy people who normally slept on their left side. When these people were made to sleep on the right side, after one week they began to show signs of sluggish digestion. When they were allowed to resume their usual left-sided sleeping position, their stomach disorders were automatically rectified.[3] Another survey of asthmatic patients showed that 7 out of 10 slept on their backs.[4] Even if you are not suffering from any chronic or acute ailment, you can avoid any forthcoming stomach or respiratory complaint by sleeping in the correct way.

Once the disorder has actually set in, a change in the flow of swara can bring some relief. If there is too much heat in the body, lying on the right side can help cool it. Conversely when the body is excessively cold, lying on the left side can help to warm it. During a fever the active pingala nostril should be purposely blocked to balance the temperature.

Before the actual onset of a disease, the flow of the swara becomes disturbed, and if this is noted beforehand, then the imbalance can be rectified and the sickness averted. For example, asthmatics feeling an attack coming on can block the active nostril to help prevent or lessen the severity of the attack. Or those who suffer from headaches should first check their digestion, and make sure that they sleep on the left side. When the headache occurs, they should then block the active nostril and stimulate the other.

20

Tattwa Vichara

Each cycle of the surya or chandra swara is affected by the pancha tattwas or five elements, which produce different types of breath by influencing the prana vayu. When a particular tattwa is active, it affects thought patterns, physical movements and capacities, interactions with other people, and all the situations of life. In order to recognize this, swara yogis practise *tattwa vichara*, the techniques of analyzing the active tattwa. Amongst all these techniques, each practitioner will find one to be the most helpful.

Each tattwa has a particular influence on the energy level of the body and mind. Therefore, by studying the predominant tattwa, the swara yogi is capable of knowing what is in store for him in certain situations. At a higher level tattwa vichara develops the pranic capacity in the chakras and aids spiritual evolution. While observing the tattwa, it can be seen that only one tattwa is active at any one time; with the advent or rise of another tattwa, the others subside. Sometimes, however, during the flow of sushumna, one tattwa is active in the right swara and another tattwa begins in the left or vice versa. This usually happens at the time of the changing swaras.

Some of the tattwas are referred to by different names but they indicate one and the same tattwa. Earth is prithvi or bhumi; water, apas or jala; fire, agni or tejas; air, vayu or pawan; ether, akasha or vyoma.

102

Each tattwa causes the air to flow out from different points of the nostrils, in a particular direction and extending to a certain distance. Prithvi flows from the centre and the air seems to come straightforward. Apas makes the breath flow slightly downward leaving the nostrils from the lower point. Agni flows from the upper point in an upward direction. Vayu flows predominantly from the outer sides and the breath can be felt moving at an angle. When akasha is active, it will seem like there is no exhalation escaping, only the warmth of the hot air will be felt on the hand.

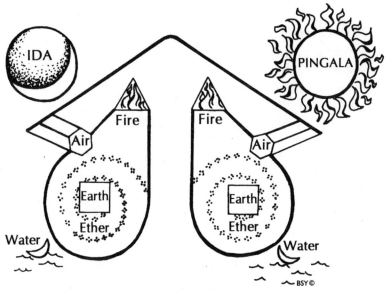

Flow of tattwas from the nose

The specific length of exhalation during each tattwa, as given in the *Shiva Swarodaya*, may vary according to the individual. This you can only find out yourself by studying your own breath.

Each tattwa also influences the flavour or taste in the mouth. Some hours after eating you can taste the distinct flavour of the prevalent tattwa.

Element	Earth	Water	Fire	Air	Ether
Length·					
in fingers	12	16	4	8	–
in inches	9	12	3	6	–
Direction of flow from the nose	centre	downwards	upwards	slanting	diffused
Duration (in minutes)	20	16	12	8	4
Sequence	3rd	4th	2nd	1st	–

- The earth element has a sweetish flavour.
- Water is astringent.
- Fire is bitter.
- Air is acidic or sour.
- Ether is pungent and hot.

If the active tattwa is not recognizable by any of these simple tests, then it can be judged by the vapour pattern formed by exhaling through the nose onto a mirror.

- If the vapour covers the mirror, earth is active.
- A half-moon shape indicates water.
- A triangular shape, fire.
- An egg or oval shape, air.
- Small dots, ether.

SHANMUKHI MUDRA
(CLOSING THE SEVEN GATES)

In order to become familiar with the nature of each tattwa and to aid recognition, the *Shiva Swarodaya* advises the practice of shanmukhi mudra.

Technique

Sit in a comfortable meditation asana, preferable siddha/siddha yoni asana or ardha/poorna padmasana.

104

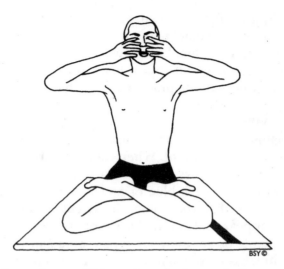

Perform shanmukhi mudra, closing only five gates: the ears, eyes and nose, with the fingers, leaving the mouth free.

Perform kaki mudra and inhale through the mouth.

While inhaling, feel the prana moving up from mooladhara to ajna chakra.

Hold the breath, performing antaranga (internal) kumbhaka and close the sixth gate (mouth) with the fingers.

Perform khechari mudra and half jalandhara bandha.

Keep the awareness at ajna.

Raise the head.

Breathe out through the nose.

Practise this five times, keeping the eyes closed. Breathe normally in between each round. When you have finished, sit quietly and look into chidakasha, the space in front of your closed eyes. See if you can perceive any colour there or a coloured circle. The colour in chidakasha will indicate the active element:

i)   Yellow indicates the presence of prithvi tattwa.

ii) White indicates apas.

iii) Red indicates agni.

iv) Blue or greyish colour, air.

v) Complete blackness or an indistinct colour of many hues, akasha. When you first begin this practice, chidakasha may still appear black afterwards, indicating inexperience in the practice rather than akasha tattwa.

Practice note

This technique requires a few months of practice before the colours become apparent. When they do start coming, the colour does not always seem distinct. Yellow is sometimes mixed with white, red, blue or any combination. It is also not necessary that the colour be circular. For example, red may appear as a triangular shape, yellow may be in a square shape, or you may see a pale blue band across the top of chidakasha. But akasha tattwa is the most difficult to perceive. It does not occur very often, and usually when it does, it is only for a very short period.

If you practise regularly twice a day, morning and evening, for six months, the colours start coming. Initially you can begin with five rounds of shanmukhi mudra. After 3–4 weeks increase to 10 rounds. Once you have perfected the practice, you will start seeing the colours before completing 10 rounds. However, it is more effective to practise in conjunction with trataka on the tattwa yantras. Then the colours may come more easily.

Yellow and red tend to appear during the day. Blue and white may come in the early morning or late evening, but yellow is most common. And if you see all the colours at once, you have found the right tattwa for spiritual experience. These are the five variations of colour. However, when the tattwas are changing, there is a period of transition during which you see a blending and combination of any nine colours or more. If you have the time and opportunity to practise three or four times a day, at the same time and on a regular basis you can make a diary of your results.

A little advice

This practice is more difficult than basic breath awareness. After your hatha yoga practices, do shanmukhi mudra, later you can do without this mudra. Concentrate on the breath which is flowing and keep on concentrating on the flow of the tattwa. When the breath is changing from the right to the left, you should know how it is changing and which tattwa is showing at the time of change.

There are a few moments when akasha tattwa, the space element, is predominant. It does not happen all the time. Sometimes this element comes with pingala, sometimes with ida, rarely with sushumna. However, when both swaras are flowing freely and there is akasha tattwa, it is time to start meditation. It will just go like a rocket. This is very momentary, maybe ten, fifteen, twenty seconds. Akasha tattwa and sushumna nadi do not usually come together, and when this happens you know it. Both the breaths are free, and the light of the tattwa is clear. At that time ask a question and it is correctly answered because that is the time of intuitive experience. If you expand that period, it is wonderful.

Influence of the tattwas in daily life

Prithvi indicates material prosperity and long-term results. Therefore, when this element is predominant, it is suggested that you do permanent, stable and quiet work, something not involving a lot of physical activity, for example, planning a building. The result will be permanent. It is also said that during prithvi, the mind becomes involved in material matters and you should involve yourself in these affairs.

Apas indicates immediate results, maybe a little less than anticipated. It also means the results are impermanent and the situation will change after some time. During apas, it is good to be engaged in calm activities involving movement. The mind tends to become involved in thoughts about the self and the physical body.

Agni gives unpleasant results. If you have planned something, it can rarely succeed. Agni is considered to be the destroyer. In fact, during agni it is advised that you keep out of harm's reach and do not voice your opinion about anything, or otherwise you will get into trouble. If you are going to burn yourself or the cooking or lose something, it happens at the time of agni tattwa. Agni also corresponds with thoughts or worries about money and valuables, etc.

Vayu, like agni, can also mean your plans will be ruined. It indicates an unstable condition. However, if you can keep your balance, everything might work out. When you are catching the train at peak hour and people are pushing you here and there, it is likely vayu will operate. Vayu also means that the mind will be self-orientated.

During akasha there are no particular thoughts or worries. You can have pleasant inner experiences and awakenings. But as far as material life and profit are concerned there cannot be any gain. So, it is better to find a quiet place, sit in a meditation pose and practise concentration and meditation.

Just as a general guideline remember that:
• Prithvi and apas are favourable in ida or pingala.
• Agni and vayu in ida signify mediocre results, but in pingala, they are destructive.
• Akasha is only beneficial if you are practising meditation or concentration.

The *Shiva Swarodaya* further states that the ideal situation is for prithvi to flow during the day and apas at night. That ensures a good balance in life and success in daily affairs.

Family planning
By utilizing the knowledge of the tattwas it is possible to know the type of child you are going to produce. According to swara yoga the result of conception is based on the active tattwa. Of course, the combination of different tattwas has different results.

Conception at the time of prithvi tattwa procures a son who will have a good financial or material position. Apas produces a girl who will also be prosperous. When agni flows through pingala, it is not an ideal time for conception because something harmful may happen to the foetus or child. In ida this effect is lessened. Vayu tattwa is also not a good time as the child may cause you some misery. During akasha it is definitely considered an inappropriate time as it indicates miscarriage or such like. But perhaps if you are a yogi, it means having a child with an awakened kundalini.

21

Tattwa Sadhana
and Chhayopasana

After developing proficiency in the art of defining the
tattwa, you can then perform trataka on the symbolic
form or yantra of each tattwa. Traditionally, these yantras
were made of specific metals and colours and inscribed with
specific mantras. Such a practice requires expert knowledge
and the swara shastras recommend the guidance of a guru in
order to perfect it. However, we can still utilize the practice
of trataka on the tattwas by drawing the yantra of each
tattwa, colouring it with the appropriate colour, and mentally
repeating the bija mantra. The yantras can be prepared
according to the charts on the following pages.

Before starting the practice, make a small dot in the
centre of the yantra so that your attention is centred and
your eyes do not waver from their point of focus. After some
practice this dot may be unnecessary.

TATTWA SADHANA

Technique

Sit in a comfortable meditation pose, back straight, head
straight, hands either in jnana mudra or chin mudra.
If the yantra is small, keep it an arm's distance away. If it
is large, adjust the position so that you can gaze without
straining. The yantra should be placed exactly at eye
level.

Qualities of the Tattwa Yantras

Element	Symbol	Dimensions	Colour of yantra	Mantra	Background
Prithvi	square	any size, equal sides	deeper shade of yellow	Lam लं	black or white
Apas	crescent moon	narrow in the middle	white	Vam वं	black
Agni	inverted triangle	equilateral	red	Ram रं	black or white
Vayu	hexagon or star	equal sides	pale blue	Yam यं	preferably black
Akash	circle	any size	small dots of many colours	Ham हं	inside yantra white, outside black

Tattwa Yantras

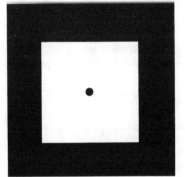

Prithvi लं

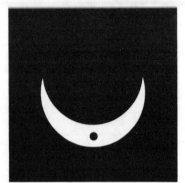

Apas वं

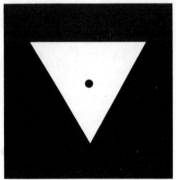

Agni रं

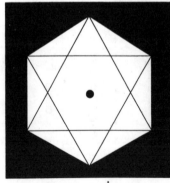

Vayu यं

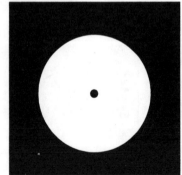

Akasha हं

BSY©

Begin with the prithvi yantra first. Practise trataka on it. The eyes should be steady.

To keep the mind quiet, mentally repeat the mantra *Lam*, keeping your gaze continually on the yantra, and your attention on the sound of the mantra. Repeat one mala of the mantra, but if the eyes become tired, close them and keep the awareness in chidakasha.

This practice should take about 5 minutes.

Then close the eyes.

Mentally visualize prithvi yantra and its colour. Repeat the same process for all the tattwa yantras.

When you have finished, remain seated and quiet. Look into chidakasha and see if there is any predominating colour or shape.

Examine the nature of your breath, its length, direction of flow, and taste the flavour in your mouth. Observe your mind, thoughts, feelings, whether you are relaxed, agitated, sleepy, hungry, anxious, etc. Now, see if you can determine the active tattwa from this analysis. If you are still unsure, perform shanmukhi mudra and go through the same process of analysis.

CHHAYOPASANA

The most significant practice of swara yoga is the art of chhayopasana. *Chhaya* means shadow, *upasana* is the practice of steady concentration. In this practice, instead of performing trataka on the yantras of the tattwas, you practise trataka on your own shadow. As a result of this practice, you can foretell from the colour and shape of the shadow, the time of death and the manner in which you will die. But, of course, this is not the ultimate intention of practising chhayopasana.

Chhayopasana is an uncomplicated but very intensive form of dharana or concentration, and it has a powerful effect on the mind. It can spontaneously arouse the state of dhyana and eventually samadhi. It is a sure way to have direct experience of *atma anubhuti*, where the atma reveals itself in a cognizable form. Therefore, chhayopasana has been a well-guarded secret throughout the ages, and its success depends purely upon the prerequisite that it is practised strictly as a sadhana under the instructions of the guru.

According to the *Shiva Swarodaya* the best time to practise is between 7–8 am. But you will have to take the time of sunrise into consideration. It means the practice should be done approximately 1–1½ hours after sunrise. It is important, however, that the sun is not very strong at the time and there are no clouds in the sky to cover it. The *Swara Chintamani* also suggests that this can be practised by moonlight on clear moonlit nights.

The *Shiva Swarodaya* says that it takes six months to become proficient in the art, whereupon you can start applying it to gain knowledge of forthcoming death.

Technique

Stand erect with your hands by your side and your back to the sun so you cast a shadow directly in front of you, either on the ground or on a plain wall.

Focus your attention and gaze on the neck region of the shadow.

Mentally repeat the mantra *Hrim Parabrahmane Namaha* 108 times.

Discontinue the practice, close the eyes for a few seconds and look into your chidakasha. You should still see the image of your shadow.

Open the eyes, and look into the sky. The image of your shadow should reappear in front of your open eyes. If it is not visible, it means you need to develop the capacity of seeing the image.

Indications from the form of the shadow

When certain parts of the body are missing from the image of your shadow, it means the following:

- Left upper arm absent: wife will die.
- Right upper arm absent: either a friend or you yourself will die.
- Arms absent: somebody close to you will become sick or pass away.
- Head missing: death will occur in one month.
- Shoulder or thigh missing: one's life will last 8 days.
- Fingers and shoulders: 6 months are left to live.
- Feet or stomach missing: death is close at hand.
- Elongated neck indicates prosperity.
- Absolutely no image of the shadow or the shadow itself is faint, then death is upon you.

The colour of the image also has to be noted:

- A black image means death will occur after 6 months or so.
- A yellow image indicates illness only.
- A red image signifies deep-rooted fear.
- A blue image means disaster is about to occur.
- Many colours all at once indicate development of psyche and intuition and perfection in yoga.

The forecasts pertaining to death should be understood as being more than just predictions. When you practise chhayopasana, you are making your mind more subtle and sensitive. The image in the sky represents your pranic body. When prana vayu does not function in any particular part of the body, it is a clear indication of disharmony in the body and that subsequent illness or even death is about to occur.

Whether or not you are interested in these matters concerning death, chhayopasana aids in removing the limitation of the finite mind. In fact, the *Shiva Swarodaya* refers to it as a method by which you can perceive the past, see more deeply into the present and know the future. In this way your whole concept of time and perception is altered.

22

The Swara Guru

In India many people still have knowledge of swara yoga. It is not difficult to get a general understanding of the science, but those who practise it are not willing to disclose their knowledge to just anyone. Even if you refer to the original texts you will have difficulty understanding the symbology and terminology used. Due to this, the Sanskrit texts are sometimes misinterpreted. So it is not completely effective to learn only from scriptural references. If you are going to delve seriously into swara yoga, it is safer and easier to try and find the guru who can initiate you into the science. This is exactly what the *Shiva Samhita* states, "Having received instructions in yoga, and having obtained a guru who knows yoga, let him practise earnestly according to the method taught by the teacher." (3:9)

However, it is very rare to find a swara guru in this modern day, and if you do, initiation is not just for anyone. This is not just for the sake of being secretive or in order to keep a valuable treasure exclusive to India alone. The sages had a very logical reason for withholding from the general public those sciences which rapidly expanded the consciousness by increasing the pranic and mental capacities.

In the past, these specific branches of tantra were kept secret because people frequently misused the techniques in order to gain greater power for selfish and destructive motives. Many suffered on account of this, but worse than

116

that the reputable science of tantra and yoga was defamed. Therefore, we should not consider any branch of the yogic science as dangerous or corrupt, but the correct purpose for which it is meant to be used must be kept in mind. For this reason since ancient times such practices as swara yoga could be learned only under the tutelage of a guru.

Inner guru

An important point arises from these considerations. What is meant by 'spiritual' intentions of swara yoga? The term 'spiritual' has nothing to do with religion or mysticism or anything in the spirit world. If your concept of spirituality has any of these connotations, then it needs some alteration. 'Spiritual' implies transformation of the lower mind so that it becomes capable of perceiving subtler and higher realms.

When the transformation occurs, experience of another all-encompassing and all-knowing mind, existing in the substratum of every living and non-living thing, is perceived. It operates something like a main radio station sending signals to smaller substations and radios. But it is only after the consciousness has undergone a certain stage of evolution that the higher mind can be realized. This is the experience of the 'inner guru'. So, if you desire to awaken the vast dormant area of your brain through swara yoga and experience the higher self, then you will have to find an evolved and enlightened person who has already undergone such an experience.

In India the guru tattwa is the most relevant part of an individual's life and sadhana. Whether your sadhana follows the lines of swara yoga or has no such formalities, the fulfilment of serving the guru is most vital.

In the tantra and yoga shastras the opening sloka always starts with an invocation to the *paramguru* (the primal and supreme guru). Of course, the name of the guru may vary depending on the era in which the text was written. Some texts refer to the paramguru as Shiva, others as Brahma or Vishnu. Nevertheless, they all indicate the one supreme

117

consciousness which pervades every aspect of creation. This invocation is intended to remind us of our ultimate existence, purpose and destiny. It does not even require faith. The mind is ever evolving. When you consciously think of the highest, purest experience, eventually your own individual consciousness will be taken into that realm where the *satguru* or true guru exists.

For people who do not have spiritual convictions and who are striving consciously to find a satisfying and permanent experience, the path of swara yoga is very effective. There are also those people who cannot accept anything other than mundane existence. These people too can practise swara yoga, because it consists of a scientific and practical system which even enables them to enjoy worldly life more fully. The *Shiva Swarodaya* clearly sums up the whole science, stating that, "It is helpful to those who are believers in a supreme being, as well as to those who are non-believers. Even to non-believers, it will give many surprises." (v. 12)

Manifestation of the guru tattwa

As the techniques start having a noticeable effect upon your whole being and your concepts of life, the purpose for which these practices are intended begins manifesting in the form of tangible experience. As swara yoga was designed to awaken the higher consciousness, whoever practises it is bound to have this experience eventually.

This system is based on scientific lines, whereby you start from a logical, comprehensive point in your physical existence and manipulate the mental and physical forces. By concentrating on the two dualistic energy forces, and eliminating all of the accumulated impurities within the energy pathways of the physical, mental and psychic bodies, the third most powerful force can be generated. That is the spiritual energy which awakens the higher faculties in the brain and consciousness.

Through swara yoga ajna chakra, or the guru chakra, is activated and for that purpose the swara shastras

118

emphasize the necessity of the external guru before the internal awakening process has begun. Thus, the *Hatha Yoga Pradipika* declares, "He who is devoted to any knowledge, while pleasing the guru with utmost attention, readily obtains the fruit of that knowledge." (3:12) Furthermore, no one can know the science better than the guru. He is fully experienced and can show you, according to your own personal development, the systematic process by which you can progress.

Therefore, even if you do not want to practise swara yoga for the realization of higher consciousness, but prefer to use it for worldly fulfilment, still it is most necessary to have a guru. He will know your inner desire and capacity, and will allow the expansion of your consciousness to proceed at a rate which you are able to handle. He knows how and for whom the practices will bring best results. Therefore, the *Shiva Samhita* states, "Only by the guru's favour is everything good relating to one's self obtained. So the guru ought to be served daily, or nothing will be auspicious." (3:14)

Shiva Swarodaya

Translation from the Original Sanskrit

Shiva Swarodaya

TRANSLATION FROM THE ORIGINAL SANSKRIT

श्री गणेशाय नम:
महेश्वरं नमस्कृत्य शैलजां गणनायकम् ।
गुरुं च परमात्मानं भजे संसारतारणम् ॥ 1 ॥

1. Having paid obeisance to Maheshwara (Lord Shiva),
Parvati and Ganesha, I bow to the guru who is verily the
supreme consciousness (Paramatma) and saviour of the
world.

श्रीदेव्युवाच
देवदेव महादेव कृपां कृत्वा ममोपरि ।
सर्वसिद्धिकरं ज्ञानं कथयस्व मम प्रभो ॥ 2 ॥

2. Devi said:
O God of Gods! Mahadeva, be gracious to me, my Lord,
and give me that knowledge which bestows perfection.

कथं ब्रह्माण्डमुत्पन्नं कथं वा परिवर्तते ।
कथं विलीयते देव वद ब्रह्माण्डनिर्णयम् ॥ 3 ॥

3. Tell me, O God, how the universe was created, how it
changes and how it dissolves – tell me that which is the
determiner of the universe.

123

ईश्वर उवाच
तत्त्वाद्ब्रह्माण्डमुत्पन्नं तत्त्वेन परिवर्तते ।
तत्त्वे विलीयते देवि तत्त्वाद्ब्रह्माण्डनिर्णय: ॥ ४ ॥

4. Ishwara said:
Creation takes place due to the tattwas (subtle essences).
It is sustained by them and finally dissolves into them.
O Devi, the tattwas are the origin of the Brahmanda
(universe).

देव्युवाच
तत्त्वमेव परं मूलं निश्चितं तत्त्ववादिभि: ।
तत्त्वस्वरूपं किं देव तत्त्वमेव प्रकाशय ॥ ५ ॥

5. Devi said:
The tattwas (elements) are the primal cause as ascertained
by the exponents of the tattwas. O Lord, what is the
nature of those elements? Kindly reveal that to me.

ईश्वर उवाच
निरञ्जनो निराकार एको देवो महेश्वर: ।
तस्मादाकाशमुत्पन्नमाकाशाद्वायु सम्भव: ॥ ६ ॥

6. Ishwara said:
There is only one birthless and formless supreme
existence from which evolves akasha (ether element),
and from akasha comes vayu (air element).

वायोस्तेजस्ततश्चापस्तत: पृथ्वीसमुद्भव: ।
एतानि पञ्चतत्त्वानि विस्तीर्णानि च पञ्चधा ॥ ७ ॥

7. From vayu originates tejas (fire element), from tejas, apas
(water element), and from apas, prithvi (earth element).
These five elements are spread throughout the whole
world in this fivefold manner.

तेभ्यो ब्रह्माण्डमुत्पन्नं तैरेव परिवर्तते ।
विलीयते च तत्रैव तत्रैव रमते पुनः ॥8॥

8. Due to these five elements creation is formed and
sustained, and again merges back into the tattwas. (This
is the continual subtle process of creation.) Thus it comes
to stay within the five elements again.

पञ्चतत्त्वमये देहे पञ्चतत्त्वानि सुन्दरि ।
सूक्ष्मरूपेण वर्तन्ते ज्ञायन्ते तत्त्वयोगिभिः ॥9॥

9. O beautiful one, the five elements are present in subtle
form within the body which originates from these five
elements. This is known by yogis who are well versed in
the science of the elements.

SWARA JNANA

अथ स्वरं प्रवक्ष्यामि शरीरस्थस्वरोदयम् ।
हंसचारस्वरूपेण भवेज्ज्ञानं त्रिकालजम् ॥10॥

10. Now I will describe the science of the origin of the
swaras which reside in the body. With the knowledge of
the swaras, which move in the form of Hamso (i.e. the
sound of the outgoing *Ham* and incoming *So* breath),
one acquires knowledge of the past, present and future.

गुह्यादगुह्यतरं सारमुपकार प्रकाशनम् ।
इदं स्वरोदयं ज्ञानं ज्ञानानां मस्तके मणिः ॥11॥

11. This science of swara is the secret of all secrets and
reveals the essence of all benefits. This science is the
crest jewel of all knowledge.

सूक्ष्मात्सूक्ष्मतरं ज्ञानं सुबोधं सत्यप्रत्ययम् ।
आश्चर्यं नास्तिके लोके आधारंत्वास्तिकेजने ॥12॥

12. This is the subtlest of subtle knowledge. It is easy to understand and is based on truth. To the atheists it is a wonder and to the theists it is the base.

DESCRIPTION OF THE DISCIPLE

शान्ते शुद्धे सदाचारे गुरुभक्त्यैकमानसे ।
दृढचित्ते कृतज्ञे च देयं चैव स्वरोदयम् ॥ 13 ॥

13. Only to one who is peaceful by nature, having pure instincts, good conduct, one-pointedness, devotion to the guru, firm determination and gratefulness, can this knowledge of swara be imparted.

दुष्टे च दुर्जने क्रुद्धे नास्तिके गुरुतल्पगे ।
हीनसत्त्वे दुराचारे स्वरज्ञानं न दीयते ॥ 14 ॥

14. This knowledge of swara should not be given to one who is wicked, villainous, angry, atheistic, of bad character, without mettle, and who commits adultery with his guru's wife.

शृणु त्वं कथितं देवि देहस्थं ज्ञानमुत्तमम् ।
येन विज्ञानमात्रेण सर्वज्ञत्वं प्रणीयते ॥ 15 ॥

15. Listen, O Goddess, as I tell you the highest knowledge situated within the body, by the mere proper knowledge of which one becomes omniscient.

स्वरे वेदाश्च शास्त्राणि स्वरे गान्धर्वमुत्तमम् ।
स्वरे च सर्वत्रैलोक्यं स्वरमात्मस्वरूपकम् ॥ 16 ॥

16. Within the swara the entire Vedas, shastras and musical knowledge are contained. Within the swara are the three planes of existence (conscious, subconscious, unconscious). Swara is verily the atma (self-illumined).

126

स्वरहीनश्च दैवज्ञो नाथहीनं यथा गृहम् ।
शास्त्रहीनं यथा वक्त्रं शिरोहीनं च यद्वपुः ॥ 17 ॥

17. Everything is meaningless without the knowledge of
swara. An astrologer without the knowledge of swara is as
useless as a masterless house, a mouth without scriptures
or a headless body.

नाडीभेदं तथा प्राणतत्त्वभेदं तथैव च ।
सुषुम्नामिश्रभेदं च यो जानाति स मुक्तिगः ॥ 18 ॥

18. The one who has discrimination regarding the nadis,
prana, tattwas and sushumna has the right to attain
liberation.

साकारे वा निराकारे शुभं वायुबलात्कृतम् ।
कथयन्ति शुभं केचित्स्वरज्ञानं वरानने ॥ 19 ॥

19. O beautiful-faced lady, either with a form or formless,
swara plays the most important role. Knowledge of the
swaras is considered to be highly auspicious.

GLORY OF THE SWARA

ब्रह्माण्ड खण्ड पिण्डाद्याः स्वरेणैव हि निर्मिताः ।
सृष्टिसंहारकर्त्ता च स्वरः साक्षान्महेश्वरः ॥ 20 ॥

20. In the macro and microcosmos all are created only by
the swara, which is also the cause of creation and
dissolution. Swara is verily Lord Shiva himself.

स्वरज्ञानात्परं गुह्यं स्वरज्ञानात्परं धनम् ।
स्वरज्ञानात्परं ज्ञानं न वा दृष्टं न वा श्रुतम् ॥ 21 ॥

21. There has neither been seen nor heard anything more
confidential, more valuable or more knowledgeable than
the knowledge of swara.

शत्रुं हन्यात्स्वरबले तथा मित्रसमागम: ।
लक्ष्मीप्राप्ति: स्वरबले कीर्ति: स्वरबले सुखम् ॥ 22 ॥

22. Through the power of the swara you can overcome the
enemy; and you can be sure to meet your friend. You can
obtain the favour of Lakshmi (the goddess of wealth and
prosperity), popularity and all sorts of pleasures.

कन्याप्राप्ति: स्वरबले स्वरतो राजदर्शनम् ।
स्वरेण देवतासिद्धि: स्वरेण क्षितिपो वश: ॥ 23 ॥

23. Through the power of swara you can obtain a wife, meet
with the great rulers and attain the perfection of the
gods. Even the most powerful ruler can be overcome by
this power.

स्वरेण गम्यते देशो भोज्यं स्वरबले तथा ।
लघुदीर्घं स्वरबले मलं चैव निवारयेत् ॥ 24 ॥

24. With the proper swara one can undertake journeys, eat
the best food, urinate and excrete.

सर्वशास्त्रपुराणादि स्मृतिवेदाङ्गपूर्वकम् ।
स्वरज्ञानात्परं तत्त्वं नास्ति किञ्चिद्द्वरानने ॥ 25 ॥

25. O lady of beautiful face, all the shastras, puranas, smritis
and the vedangas are nothing beyond the knowledge of
swara.

नामरूपादिका: सर्वे मिथ्या सर्वेषु विभ्रम: ।
अज्ञानमोहिता मूढा यावत्तत्त्वं न विद्यते ॥ 26 ॥

26. Unless you know about the tattwas, you are under the
illusion of name and form, and ignorance itself keeps
you in the dark.

इदं स्वरोदयं शास्त्रं सर्वशास्त्रोत्तमोत्तमम् ।
आत्मघटप्रकाशार्थं प्रदीपकलिकोपमम् ॥ 27 ॥

27. The Swarodaya shastra is the best of all scriptures, and like a jyoti it is capable of lighting the house of your own spirit.

यस्मै कस्मै परस्मै वा न प्रोक्तं प्रश्नहेतवे ।
तस्मादेतत्स्वयं ज्ञेयमात्मनोवाऽऽत्मनात्मनि ॥ 28 ॥

28. This teaching should not be revealed simply to answer someone's questions, but it should be mastered for one's own self, by one's own intellect, in one's own body.

न तिथिर्न च नक्षत्रं न वारो ग्रहदेवता ।
न च विष्टिर्व्यतीपातो वैधृत्याद्यास्तथैव च ॥ 29 ॥

29. If you have knowledge of the swara, it is not necessary to consult the date, stars, days, planets, gods, conjunction of the stars or disorders of the humors (phlegm, bile, wind) before starting any project.

कुयोगो नास्त्यतो देवि भविता वा कदाचन ।
प्राप्ते स्वरबले शुद्धे सर्वमेव शुभं फलम् ॥ 30 ॥

30. O Goddess, neither had there ever been nor would there ever be an inauspicious moment when the pure strength of the swaras is available, because in that case all results would be auspicious.

ABOUT THE NADIS

देहमध्ये स्थिता नाड्यो बहुरूपाः सुविस्तराः ।
ज्ञातव्याश्च बुधैर्नित्यं स्वदेहज्ञानहेतवे ॥ 31 ॥

31. In this body there are many forms of nadis which extend throughout. The wise must always know them for true understanding of their own body.

नाभिस्थानात्स्कन्धोर्ध्वमङ्कुराइव निर्गता: ।
द्विसप्ततिसहस्राणि देहमध्ये व्यवस्थिता: ॥ 32 ॥

32. Originating like sprouts from the navel region, these
    nadis extend up to the shoulders. There are seventy-two
    thousand of them spread throughout the body.

नाडीस्था कुण्डलीशक्तिर्भुजंगाकारशायिनी ।
ततो दशोर्ध्वगा नाड्योदशैवाध: प्रतिष्ठिता: ॥ 33 ॥

33. Kundalini shakti exists in these nadis, lying in the
    form of a snake. Ten nadis extend upwards and ten
    downwards.

द्वे द्वे तिर्यग्गते नाड्यौ चतुर्विंशतिसंख्यया ।
प्रधाना दशनाड्यस्तु दश वायुप्रवाहिका: ॥ 34 ॥

34. On each side are two nadis, both going in oblique
    directions. In this manner there are twenty-four nadis of
    which ten are significant for the transition of ten vayus.

तिर्यगूर्ध्वास्तथानाड्यो वायुदेहसमन्विता: ।
चक्रवत्संस्थिता देहे सर्वे: प्राणसमाश्रिता: ॥ 35 ॥

35. From every angle, up and down, all these nadis join like
    a wheel, but they are all under the control of the one
    prana.

तासां मध्ये दश श्रेष्ठा दशानां तिस्र उत्तमा: ।
इडा च पिंगला चैव सुषुम्ना च तृतीयका ॥ 36 ॥

36. Of all the nadis, ten are prominent. Of the ten, ida,
    pingala and sushumna are most important.

गान्धारी हस्तिजिह्वा च पूषा चैव यशस्विनी ।
अलम्बुषा कुहूश्चैव शङ्खिनी दशमी तथा ॥ 37 ॥

37. The others are gandhari, hastijihva, poosha, yashaswini, alambusha, kuhu and the tenth is shankhini.

PLACEMENT OF THE NADIS

इडा वामे स्थिता भागे पिंगला दक्षिणे स्मृता ।
सुषुम्ना मध्यदेशे तु गान्धारी वामचक्षुषि ॥ 38 ॥

38. Ida nadi is on the left side of the body, pingala on the right side, sushumna in the centre, and gandhari in the left eye.

दक्षिणे हस्तिजिह्वा च पूषा कर्णे च दक्षिणे ।
यशस्विनी वामकर्णे आनने चाप्यलम्बुषा ॥ 39 ॥

39. Hastijihva is in the right eye, poosha in the right ear, yashaswini in the left ear, alambusha in the mouth.

कुहूश्च लिङ्गदेशे तु मूलस्थाने तु शङ्खिनी ।
एवं द्वारं समाश्रित्य तिष्ठन्ति दशनाडिका: ॥ 40 ॥

40. Kuhu is in the reproductive organs and shankhini in the anal region. In this manner all these ten nadis are situated in the openings of the body.

पिङ्गलेडा सुषुम्ना च प्राणमार्गे समाश्रिता: ।
एताहि दशनाड्यस्तु देहमध्ये व्यवस्थिता: ॥ 41 ॥

41. The three main channels, ida, pingala and sushumna, are located in the pranic passage. These ten nadis are arranged inside the body.

नामानि नाडिकानां तु वातानां तु वदाम्यहम् ।
प्राणोऽपान: समानश्च उदानोव्यान एव च ॥ 42 ॥

42. I have told you the names of the nadis, now I will tell you the names of the vayus related to the nadis. They are prana, apana, samana, udana and vyana.

नाग: कूर्मोऽथ कृकलो देवदत्तो धनञ्जय: ।
हृदि प्राणो वसेन्नित्यमपानो गुदमण्डले ॥43॥

43. And naga, kurma, krikara, devadatta, dhananjaya are the
subsidiary pranas. The eternal prana exists in the heart
and apana vayu is in the excretory organs.

समानो नाभिदेशे तु उदान: कण्ठमध्यग: ।
व्यानो व्यापी शरीरेषु प्रधाना: दश वायव: ॥44॥

44. Samana is situated in the navel region. Udana is in the
throat. Vyana pervades the whole body. Like this ten
vayus are prominent.

प्राणाद्या: पञ्च विख्याता नागाद्या: पञ्च वायव: ।
तेषामपि च पञ्चानां स्थानानि च वदाम्यहम् ॥45॥

45. I told you the five main pranas, now I will tell you the
other five vayus such as naga, etc. and their places.

उद्गारे नाग आख्यात: कूर्म उन्मीलने स्मृत: ।
कृकल: क्षुतकृतज्ञेयो देवदत्तो विजृम्भणे ॥46॥

46. Naga vayu is for vomiting and belching; kurma for
opening and closing the eyes and blinking; krikara for
sneezing; devadatta for yawning.

न जहाति मृतं वापि सर्वव्यापी धनञ्जय: ।
एते नाडीषु सर्वासु भ्रमन्ते जीवरूपिण: ॥47॥

47. The dhananjaya vayu, which pervades the entire body,
does not leave the body even after death. In this manner,
the ten vayus roam in the body of the living being
through all these nadis.

प्रकटं प्राणसञ्चारं लक्षयेद्देहमध्यत: ।
इडापिङ्गलासुषुम्नाभिर्नाडीभिस्तिसृभिर्बुध: ॥48॥

48. The wise should clearly understand the movement of the prana within the body through the three nadis, ida, pingala and sushumna.

इडा वामे च विज्ञेया पिङ्गला दक्षिणे स्मृता ।
इडानाडीस्थिता वामा ततो व्यस्ता च पिङ्गला ॥ 49 ॥

49. Ida should be known to be situated on the left side (of the spinal cord) and pingala on the right, criss-crossing each other.

इडायां तु स्थितश्चन्द्रः पिङ्गलायां च भास्करः ।
सुषुम्ना शम्भुरूपेण शम्भुर्हंसस्वरूपतः ॥ 50 ॥

50. The moon is situated in ida nadi and the sun in pingala nadi. Shiva is in sushumna nadi in the form of Hamsa (i.e. the sound of the outgoing *Ham* and incoming *Sa* breath).

हकारो निर्गमे प्रोक्तः सकारेण प्रवेशनम् ।
हकारः शिवरूपेण सकारः शक्तिरुच्यते ॥ 51 ॥

51. It is said that when you exhale, the sound is *Ha* and when you inhale the sound is *Sa*. *Ha* is in the form of Shiva (consciousness) and *Sa* is in the form of Shakti (energy).

शक्तिरूपः स्थितश्चन्द्रो वामनाडीप्रवाहकः ।
दक्षनाडीप्रवाहश्च शम्भुरूपो दिवाकरः ॥ 52 ॥

52. The controller of the flow of the left nadi is the moon who also resides in it in the form of Shakti. The controller of the flow of the right nadi is the sun in the form of Shambhu (Shiva).

श्वासे सकारसंस्थे तु यद्दानं दीयते बुधैः ।
तद्दानं जीवलोकेऽस्मिन् कोटिकोटिगुणं भवेत् ॥ 53 ॥

53. If a wise man performs an act of charity at the time of inhalation, it bestows upon him a millionfold auspicious fruits in this very lifetime.

YOGA SADHANA

अनेन लक्षयेद्योगी चैकचित्तः समाहितः ।
सर्वमेवविजानीयान्मार्गे वै चन्द्रसूर्ययोः ॥ ५४ ॥

54. Through one-pointed awareness, the yogi becomes alert. In this way the yogi is able to know everything by the activities of his lunar and solar nadis.

ध्यायेत्तत्त्वं स्थिरे जीवे अस्थिरे न कदाचन ।
इष्टसिद्धिर्भवेत्तस्य महालाभो जयस्तथा ॥ ५५ ॥

55. Only when the mind is one-pointed and steady should one concentrate on the tattwa, but never when the mind is distracted. Then one can obtain the desired goal, great gain and victory.

चन्द्रसूर्यसमभ्यासं ये कुर्वन्ति सदा नराः ।
अतीतानागतज्ञानं तेषां हस्तगतं भवेत् ॥ ५६ ॥

56. Those who always practise thoroughly controlling their lunar and solar nadis have knowledge of past and future ready at hand.

वामे चामृतरूपा स्याज्जगदाप्यायनं परम् ।
दक्षिणे चरभागेन जगदुत्पादयेत्सदा ॥ ५७ ॥

57. Ida nadi on the left is like amrit (nectar) and the giver of strength and nourishment. Pingala on the right is responsible for all creativity.

मध्यमा भवति क्रूरा दुष्टा सर्वत्र कर्मसु ।
सर्वत्र शुभकार्येषु वामा भवति सिद्धिदा ॥ ५८ ॥

58. The middle channel (sushumna) is cruel and wicked in all activities. In all kinds of auspicious affairs, the left channel (ida) always gives success.

निर्गमे तु शुभा वामा प्रवेशे दक्षिणा शुभा ।
चन्द्र: सम:सुविज्ञेयो रविस्तु विषम: सदा ॥ 59 ॥

59. When you leave the house, it is auspicious if the left nadi is flowing. At the time of entering, it is auspicious when the right flows. The lunar nadi is smooth and virtuous and surya is always rough and non-virtuous.

चन्द्र: स्त्री पुरुष: सूर्यश्चन्द्रो गौरोऽसितो रवि: ।
चन्द्रनाडीप्रवाहेण सौम्यकार्याणि कारयेत् ॥ 60 ॥

60. Chandra, the lunar flow, is the female principle; and surya, the solar flow, is the male principle. Understand that the moon is Shakti, the sun is Shiva. The complexion of the moon is fair and that of the sun is dark. During the flow of chandra nadi (ida), placid works should be done.

सूर्यनाडी प्रवाहेण रौद्रकर्माणि कारयेत् ।
सुषुम्नाया: प्रवाहेण भुक्तिमुक्तिफलानि च ॥ 61 ॥

61. During the flow of surya nadi, difficult and hard works should be done. During the flow of sushumna those actions leading to bhukti (sensual enjoyment) and mukti (liberation) should be undertaken.

आदौ चन्द्र: सिते पक्षे भास्करो हि सितेतरे ।
प्रतिपत्तो दिनान्याहुस्त्रीणित्रीणि कृतोदये ॥ 62 ॥

62. During the first three days of the bright fortnight, the lunar nadi flows first and then alternates. In the first three days of the dark fortnight, the solar nadi flows first and then alternates. From this order you should know the rising time of the swara.

सार्धद्विघटिके ज्ञेय: शुक्ले कृष्णे शशी रवि: ।
वहत्येकदिनेनैव यथा षष्टिघटी: क्रमात् ॥ ६३ ॥

63. Beginning with the lunar swara in the bright fortnight
and the solar swara in the dark fortnight these swaras
alternate during twenty-four hours of the day and night
at the frequency of two and a half ghatis (sixty minutes)
each (i.e. each swara alternates twenty-four times in one
day and night).

वहेयुस्तद्घटीमध्ये पञ्चतत्त्वानि निर्दिशेत् ।
प्रतिपत्तो दिनान्याहुर्विपरीते विवर्जयेत् ॥ ६४ ॥

64. It should be understood that in each hour the five tattwas
are active. From the first three days, if the opposite nadi
is active, auspicious work should not be attempted.

शुक्लपक्षे भवेद्वामा कृष्णपक्षे च दक्षिणा ।
जानीयात्प्रतिपत्पूर्वं योगी तद्घतमानस: ॥ ६५ ॥

65. From the first day of the bright fortnight the left swara
should flow, and in the dark fortnight from the first
day the right swara. Then the yogi should perform the
right actions with a concentrated mind, and he will be
successful.

शशाङ्कं वारयेद्रात्रौ दिवा वारय च भास्करम् ।
इत्यभ्यासरतो नित्यं स योगी नात्र संशय: ॥ ६६ ॥

66. In the night the lunar swara should be suppressed and
in the day the solar. The person who practises this daily
is a perfected yogi, there is no doubt.

सूर्येण बध्यते सूर्यश्चन्द्रश्चन्द्रेण बध्यते ।
यो जानाति क्रियामेतां त्रैलोक्यं वशगं क्षणात् ॥ ६७ ॥

67. Through pingala the sun can be controlled, and through ida the moon can be controlled. The one who knows this process has the power of the three worlds in a moment.

उदयं चन्द्रमार्गेण सूर्यणास्तमनं यदि ।
तदा ते गुणसंघाता विपरीतं विवर्जयेत् ॥ 68 ॥

68. When the cycle begins with the lunar swara at sunrise and ends in the solar swara at sunset, then there is merit in gaining property, but if the opposite occurs, avoid it.

DESCRIPTION OF THE AUSPICIOUS/INAUSPICIOUS NADIS ACCORDING TO THE DAY

गुरुशुक्रबुधेन्दूनां वासरे वामनाडिका ।
सिद्धिदा सर्वकार्येषु शुक्लपक्षे विशेषतः ॥ 69 ॥

69. The actions done on Wednesday, Thursday, Friday and Monday when the left swara flows, are most fruitful, especially during the bright fortnight.

अर्काङ्गारकसौरीणां वासरे दक्षनाडिका ।
स्मर्त्तव्या चरकार्येषु कृष्णपक्षे विशेषतः ॥ 70 ॥

70. When the right swara flows on Sunday, Tuesday and Saturday, whatever roving business is done happens to be most prosperous, especially during the dark fortnight.

RULES OF THE FIVE TATTWAS

प्रथमं वहते वायुर्द्वितीयं च तथाऽनल: ।
तृतीयं वहते भूमिश्चतुर्थं वारुणो वहेत् ॥ 71 ॥

71. During the flow of the swara, first the air element is active, then fire, then earth, water and ether.

सार्द्धद्विघटिके पञ्च क्रमेणैवोदयन्ति च ।
क्रमादेकैकनाड्यां च तत्त्वानां पृथगुद्भव: ॥ 72 ॥

72. During the period of two and a half ghatis (i.e. one hour), the five elements are active in this order. The elements arise separately in the flow of each nadi.

ZODIAC SIGNS ACCORDING TO THE DAY AND NIGHT

अहोरात्रस्य मध्ये तु ज्ञेया द्वादशसंक्रमा: ।
बृषकर्कटकन्यालिमृगमीना   निशाकरे ॥ 73 ॥

73. During the period of one day and night (i.e. twenty-four hours), twelve zodiac transitions occur. Taurus, Cancer, Virgo, Scorpio, Capricorn and Pisces transit in the lunar swara.

मेषसिंहौ च कुम्भश्च तुला च मिथुनं धनुम् ।
उदये   दक्षिणे   ज्ञेय: शुभाशुभविनिर्णय: ॥ 74 ॥

74. Aries, Leo, Aquarius, Libra, Gemini and Sagittarius transit in the solar swara. Thus, one should determine the auspicious and inauspicious nature of events from the rising of the zodiacal signs.

138

तिष्ठेत्पूर्वोत्तरे चन्द्रो भानुः पश्चिमदक्षिणे ।
दक्षनाड्याः प्रसारे तु न गच्छेद्याम्यपश्चिमे ॥ ७५ ॥

75. The lunar swara represents the east and north and the
solar swara the west and south. When the solar swara
flows, one should not go towards the south and west.

वामाचार प्रवाहे तु न गच्छेत्पूर्वउत्तरे ।
परिपन्थिभयं तस्य गतोऽसौ न निवर्त्तते ॥ ७६ ॥

76. During the flow of the lunar swara, one should not go
towards the north and east as there is an apprehension
of violence from the enemy or the robber and perhaps
one may never come back.

तत्र तस्मान्न गन्तव्यं बुधैः सर्वहितैषिभिः ।
तदा तत्र तु संयाते मृत्युरेव न संशयः ॥ ७७ ॥

77. Therefore, the wise who are the well-wishers of everyone
should not go in the directions prohibited above. If they
go, they may meet with death. There is no doubt about
it.

शुक्लपक्षे द्वितीयायामर्के वहति चन्द्रमाः ।
दृश्यतेलाभदः पुंसां सौख्यं प्रजायते ॥ ७८ ॥

78. If, on the second day of the bright fortnight, the lunar
swara is flowing when the solar swara should flow, it is
beneficial. One experiences much pleasure and enjoyment throughout the lunar flow.

सूर्योदये यदा सूर्यश्चन्द्रश्चन्द्रोदये भवेत् ।
सिध्यन्ति सर्वकार्याणि दिवारात्रिगतान्यपि ॥ ७९ ॥

79. If the solar swara flows at sunrise, and the lunar swara flows at moonrise, all sorts of actions undertaken at any time will prosper on that day.

चन्द्रकाले यदा सूर्यश्चन्द्र: सूर्योदये भवेत् ।
उद्वेग: कलहो हानि: शुभं सर्वं निवारयेत् ॥ 80 ॥

80. But if the solar swara is active at moonrise and the lunar swara at sunrise, there will be tension, conflict and loss. Do not undertake auspicious activities at this time.

सूर्यस्य वाहे प्रवदन्ति विज्ञा ज्ञानं ह्यगम्यस्य तु निश्चयेन ।
श्वासेन युक्तस्य तु शीतरश्मे: प्रवाहकाले फलमन्यथा स्यात् ॥ 81 ॥

81. The wise say that during the flow of the solar swara one can certainly obtain knowledge of subtle or inaccessible things; while under the flow of the lunar swara, the results are reversed.

DESCRIPTIONS OF THE REVERSE SITUATION

यदा प्रत्यूषकालेन विपरीतोदयो भवेत् ।
चन्द्रस्थाने वहत्यर्को रविस्थाने च चन्द्रमा: ॥ 82 ॥

82. If in the morning the opposite swara flows (i.e. if the solar swara flows instead of the lunar or the lunar flows instead of the solar), these are the results:

प्रथमे तु मनोद्वेगं धनहानिर्द्वितीयके ।
तृतीये गमनं प्रोक्तमिष्टनाशं चतुर्थके ॥ 83 ॥

83. In the first period, fickleness of mind; in the second, loss of wealth; in the third, travel or movement; in the fourth, destruction of cherished things.

पञ्चमे राज्यविध्वंसं षष्ठे सर्वार्थनाशनम् ।
सप्तमे व्याधिदु:खानि अष्टमे मृत्युमादिशेत् ॥ 84 ॥

84. In the fifth, collapse of the state (or home); in the sixth, destruction of all valuables; in the seventh, sickness and suffering; in the eighth, death.

कालत्रये दिनान्यष्ट विपरीतं यदा वहेत् ।
तदा दुष्टफलं प्रोक्तं किञ्चिन्न्यूनं तु शोभनम् ॥ 85 ॥

85. If the opposite swara flows for eight days in all three periods (i.e. in the morning, at noon and at night), then bad results will occur. A little reduction in the irregularity will be fortunate.

प्रातर्मध्याह्नयोश्चन्द्रः सायंकाले दिवाकरः ।
तदा नित्यं जयो लाभो विपरीतं विवर्जयेत् ॥ 86 ॥

86. If the lunar swara flows in the morning and afternoon, and the solar swara in the evening, there will be victory and gain. In the reverse situation avoid everything.

वामे वा दक्षिणे वापि यत्र संक्रमते शिवः ।
कृत्वा तत्पादमादौ च यात्रा भवति सिद्धिदा ॥ 87 ॥

87. Step forward with the foot that corresponds to the active swara; this brings success on the journey.

चन्द्रः समपदः कार्यो रविस्तु विषमः सदा ।
पूर्णपादं पुरस्कृत्य यात्रा भवति सिद्धिदा ॥ 88 ॥

88. During the lunar swara take an even number of steps forward, and during the solar swara an uneven number. That ensures a prosperous journey and yatra siddhi (success of travel).

FULFILMENT OF DESIRES

यत्राङ्गे वहते वायुस्तदङ्गकरसन्तलात् ।
सुप्तोत्थितो मुखं स्पृष्ट्वा लभते वाञ्छितं फलम् ॥ 89 ॥

89. By touching the mouth with the palm of the hand which is on the side of the active swara, when rising in the morning, one achieves one's desired goal.

परदत्ते तथा ग्राह्यो गृहान्निर्गमनेऽपि च ।
यदङ्गे वहते नाडी ग्राह्यं तेन करांघ्रिणा ॥ 90 ॥

90. When giving or receiving or going out of one's house, one should use the hand or foot which is on the side of the active swara.

न हानि: कलहो नैव कण्टकैनार्पि भिद्यते ।
निवर्तते सुखी चैव सर्वोपद्रववर्जित: ॥ 91 ॥

91. By following this advice one will remain free from loss, conflict and trouble from enemies. One will also be free from all troubles and return home happily.

गुरुबन्धुनृपामात्येष्वन्येषु शुभदायिनी ।
पूर्णाङ्गे खलु कर्तव्या कार्यसिद्धिर्मन: स्थिता ॥ 92 ॥

92. For fulfilment of auspicious desires by the gurus (elders), relatives, kings, ministers and others, keep them on the side of the active swara (at the time of meeting).

अरिचौराधर्मधर्मा अन्येषां वादिनिग्रह: ।
कर्तव्या: खलु रिक्तायां जयलाभसुखार्थिभि: ॥ 93 ॥

93. If you want to overcome and punish an enemy, a thief, a person committing unrighteous deeds, an opponent, etc., keep them on the side of the non-active swara. To overcome all these and obtain pleasure, you should act in such a manner.

दूरदेशे विधातव्यं गमनं तु हिमद्युतौ ।
अभ्यर्णदेशे दीप्ते तु करणमिति केचन ॥ ९४ ॥

94. According to some people one should travel to a distant place during the flow of the lunar swara and to a nearby place during the flow of the solar swara.

यत्किञ्चित्पूर्वमुद्दिष्टं लाभादि समरागमः ।
तत्सर्वं पूर्णनाडीषु जायते निर्विकल्पकम् ॥ ९५ ॥

95. Whatever has been said earlier about accumulation of profits, wars and battles, etc., all that happens beyond doubt when the swaras are flowing in their full strength.

शून्यनाड्या विपर्यस्तं यत्पूर्वं प्रतिपादितं ।
जायते नान्यथा चैव यथा सर्वज्ञभाषितम् ॥ ९६ ॥

96. The results of the actions which have been explained earlier are surely reversed if they are undertaken with the closed nadi, as has been said by the omniscient one (i.e. Lord Shiva).

व्यवहारे खलोच्चाटे द्वेषिविद्यादिवञ्चके ।
कुपितस्वामिचौराद्ये पूर्णस्थाः स्युर्भयङ्कराः ॥ ९७ ॥

97. When the swara is in full flow, there will be a frightful outcome in performing activities like extradition of the wicked, dealing with an enemy, a thief, a destroyer of right knowledge and in facing an angry master.

दूराध्वनि शुभश्चन्द्रो निर्विघ्नोऽभीष्टसिद्धिदः ।
प्रवेशकार्यहेतौ च सूर्यनाडीप्रशस्यते ॥ ९८ ॥

98. On a long journey the lunar swara is fruitful and gives the desired siddhi (perfection) without obstacle, but for entering the house, the solar nadi is auspicious.

अयोग्ये योग्यता नाड्या योग्यस्थानेप्ययोग्यता ।
कार्यानुबन्धनो जीवो यथा रुद्रस्तथाचरेत् ॥ 99 ॥

99. (The favourable flow of) the swara grants capability to
an incapable person whereas it (an unfavourable swara)
makes even a capable person incapable. Since all living
entities are bound by the reaction of their karma, one
should act according to one's swara.

चन्द्राचारे विषहते सूर्यो बलिवशं नयेत् ।
सुषुम्नायां भवेन्मोक्ष एको देवस्त्रिधा स्थितः ॥ 100 ॥

100. The active lunar swara takes away poison and the solar
swara flow brings the powerful under control. Moksha
is achieved during the flow of sushumna. Thus, one
god (swara) has a threefold existence.

शुभान्यशुभकार्याणि क्रियन्तेऽहर्निशं यदा ।
तदाकार्यानुरोधेन कार्यं नाडीप्रचालनम् ॥ 101 ॥

101. When one has to perform auspicious and inauspicious
works day and night, then one should make the swara
flow according to the demand of the work.

AUSPICIOUS ACTS DURING
THE FLOW OF IDA NADI

स्थिरकर्मण्यलङ्कारे दूराध्वगमने तथा ।
आश्रमे धर्मप्रासादे वस्तूनां संग्रहेऽपि च ॥ 102 ॥

102. Stable or permanent actions, purchasing jewellery,
undertaking a long journey, constructing an ashram or
temple, collecting things.

वापीकूपतडागादेः प्रतिष्ठा स्तम्भदेवयोः ।
यात्रा दाने विवाहे च वस्त्रालङ्कार भूषणे ॥ 103 ॥

103. Digging small or big wells and ponds, consecrating the idol of a deity, making a journey, donating, arranging marriages and acquiring clothes, ornaments and decorative articles.

शान्तिके पौष्टिके चैव दिव्यौषधिरसायने ।
स्वस्वामिदर्शने मित्रे वाणिज्येकणसंग्रहे ॥ 104 ॥

104. Doing peaceful work, obtaining nourishment, taking divine medicines and chemicals, meeting one's master, making friends, doing commercial business, collecting grain.

गृहप्रवेशे सेवायां कृषौ च बीजवापने ।
शुभकर्मणि सन्धौ च निर्गमे च शुभ: शशी ॥ 105 ॥

105. Entering a new house, doing service, farming, sowing seeds, performing auspicious works, forming an alliance and going out; these are the best actions to perform during the flow of the left swara.

विद्यारम्भादिकार्येषु बान्धवानां च दर्शने ।
जन्ममोक्षे च धर्मे च दीक्षायां मन्त्रसाधने ॥ 106 ॥

106. Beginning studies, meeting friends and relatives, birth and death, performing religious rites, taking initiation and practising one's mantra.

कालविज्ञानसूत्रे तु चतुष्पादगृहागमे ।
कालव्याधिचिकित्सायां स्वामिसम्बोधने तथा ॥ 107 ॥

107. Reading sutras about the science of time (past, present and future), bringing cattle to the home, treating incurable diseases, addressing one's master.

गजाश्वारोहणे धन्विगजाश्वानां च बन्धने ।
परोपकरणे चैव निधीनां स्थापने तथा ॥108॥

108. Mounting an elephant or horse, and keeping the horse
or elephant in the stable, practising archery, performing
charity and serving others, keeping wealth in security.

गीतावाद्यादिनृत्यादौ नृत्यशास्त्रविचारणे ।
पुरग्रामनिवेशे च तिलकक्षेत्रधारणे ॥109॥

109. Singing, playing music, dancing and studying the art
of dancing, entering a city or a village, applying tilak,
and acquiring land.

आर्तिशोकविषादेषु ज्वरितेमूर्च्छितऽपि वा ।
स्वजनस्वामिसम्बन्धे अन्नादेर्दारुसंग्रहे ॥110॥

110. Helping those with acute sufferings, who have fever or
are in an unconscious state, interacting with relatives
and one's master, collecting wood and grains.

स्त्रीणां दन्तादिभूषायां वृष्टेरागमने तथा ।
गुरुपूजाविषादीनां चालने च वरानने ॥111॥

111. O Beautiful Parvati, it is also good for women's dental
decoration, the arrival of rain, worship of the guru and
counteracting poison.

इडायां सिद्धिदं प्रोक्तं योगाभ्यासादि कर्म च ।
तत्रापि वर्जयेद्वायुं तेज आकाशमेव च ॥112॥

112. It is said ida brings perfection in all actions, like the
practice of yoga. But avoid the three elements air, fire,
and ether.

सर्वकार्याणि सिद्ध्यन्ति दिवारात्रिगतान्यपि ।
सर्वेषु शुभकार्येषु चन्द्रचार: प्रशस्यते ॥113॥

113. All works, whether done during the day or night, are successful while the lunar swara (ida nadi) is flowing. In fact, the flow of the moon is favourable for all auspicious works.

SUCCESSFUL ACTS DURING
THE FLOW OF PINGALA NADI

कठिनक्रूरविद्यानां पठने पाठने तथा ।
स्त्रीसंगवेश्यागमने महानौकाधिरोहणे ॥ 114 ॥

114. Learning or teaching difficult and cruel vidyas (maran, mohan, vashikaran, etc.), interacting with women, prostitution, boarding a ship.

भ्रष्टकार्ये सुरापाने वीरमन्त्राद्युपासने ।
विह्वलोद्ध्वंसदेशादौ विषदाने च वैरिणाम् ॥ 115 ॥

115. All the worst and meanest actions like drinking wine, practising difficult (vir) mantras and such forms of upasana, being in a state of unrest, destroying the country and poisoning the enemy.

शास्त्राभ्यासे च गमने मृगयापशुविक्रये ।
इष्टिकाकाष्ठपाषाणरत्नघर्षणदारणे ॥ 116 ॥

116. Studying the scriptures, travelling, hunting, selling cattle, making bricks, breaking stones, cutting wood and grinding or polishing gems.

गत्यभ्यासे यन्त्रतन्त्रे दुर्गपर्वतरोहणे ।
द्यूते चौर्ये गजाश्वादिरथसाधनवाहने ॥ 117 ॥

117. Speeding, learning about yantra and tantra, scaling a fort or mountain, gambling, stealing, controlling an elephant, horse, chariot or other conveyance.

व्यायामे मारणोच्चाटे षट्कर्मादिकसाधने ।
यक्षिणीयक्षवेतालविषभूतादि   निग्रहे ॥ 118 ॥

118. Exercising (gymnastics), performing tantric acts like
maran and uchattan (killing and ruining an enemy by
magic spells), practising the shatkarmas, overcoming
the powers of yaksha and yakshini (demigods), vetal
(ghosts) and poisonous creatures.

खरोष्ट्रमहिषादीनां गजाश्वारोहणे तथा ।
नदीजलौघतरणे   भेषजे   लिपिलेखने ॥ 119 ॥

119. Riding a donkey, camel, buffalo, horse or elephant,
swimming across a river or in the sea, healing and
using medicines, writing letters.

मारणे मोहने स्तम्भे विद्वेषोच्चाटने वशे ।
प्रेरणे कर्षणे क्षोभे दाने च क्रयविक्रये ॥ 120 ॥

120. Killing, attracting, fascinating, paralyzing others,
causing hatred amongst others, enchanting and
inspiring others, cultivating, donating, being enraged
and disturbed and buying and selling.

प्रेताकर्षणविद्वेषे   शत्रुनिग्रहणेऽपि   च ।
खड्गहस्ते वैरियुद्धे भोगे वा राजदर्शने ।
भोज्ये स्नाने व्यवहारे दीप्तकार्ये रवि: शुभ: ॥ 121 ॥

121. The solar swara is auspicious for attracting (calling)
spirits, hostility, killing the enemy, using the sword
while fighting the enemy, sensual pleasure, having an
audience with the king, eating and feasting, bathing,
general dealings and accomplishing outstanding deeds.

भुक्तमार्गे च मन्दाग्नौ स्त्रीणां वश्यादिकर्मणि ।
शयनं सूर्यवाहेन कर्तव्यं सर्वदा बुधै: ॥ 122 ॥

148

122. The wise should always do the following activities during the flow of the solar swara: eating, gratifying the senses, stimulating the appetite, captivating women and going to bed.

क्रूराणि सर्वकर्माणि चराणि विविधानि च ।
तानि सिद्ध्यन्ति सूर्येण नात्रकार्यविचारणा ॥ 123 ॥

123. All cruel and harsh works, and various types of works requiring dynamism are successful during the flow of the solar swara. There should not be a second thought about it.

CHARACTERISTICS OF SUSHUMNA NADI

क्षणं वामे क्षणं दक्षे यदा वहति मारुत: ।
सुषुम्ना सा च विज्ञेया सर्वकार्यहरा स्मृता ॥ 124 ॥

124. If the left swara flows one moment and the right the next (if you cannot decide whether it is ida or pingala), know sushumna is flowing. At this time no action can give worldly profit. Shoonya swara destroys all actions (arouses non-attachment).

तस्यां नाड्यां स्थितो वह्निर्ज्वलते कालरूपक: ।
विषवत्तं   विजानीयात्सर्वकार्यविनाशनम् ॥ 125 ॥

125. The fire element residing in the sushumna nadi burns like the fire of destruction and one should know this fire to be a poison and destroyer of all actions.

यदानुक्रममुल्लंघ्य यस्यनाडीद्वयं वहेत् ।
तदा तस्य विजानीयादशुभं नात्र संशय: ॥ 126 ॥

126. When both the nadis (ida and pingala) flow in a person transgressing their sequences, then it is inauspicious for him. There is no doubt about it.

क्षणं वामे क्षणं दक्षे विषमं भावमादिशेत् ।
विपरीतं फलं ज्ञेयं ज्ञातव्यं च वरानने ॥ 127 ॥

127. If in one moment the breath flows through the left
swara and the next moment through the right swara, it
should be considered to be irregular; and O fair-faced
goddess, the reverse results then occur.

उभयोरेव सञ्चरं विषवत्तं विदुर्बुधाः ।
न कुर्यात्क्रूरसौम्यानि तत्सर्वं विफलं भवेत् ॥ 128 ॥

128. According to the wise, when both the nadis flow
together, it is like poison. All actions good or bad
should be avoided because whatever work is done gives
no result.

जीविते मरणे प्रश्ने लाभालाभे जयाजये ।
विषमे विपरीते च संस्मरेज्जगदीश्वरम् ॥ 129 ॥

129. There is no alternative but to pray to God if the question
of life or death, profit or loss, victory or defeat arises, or
if one has to face an odd or adverse situation during the
flow of sushumna.

ईश्वरे चिन्तिते कार्यं योगाभ्यासादि कर्म च ।
अन्यत्तत्र न कर्त्तव्यं जयलाभसुखैषिभिः ॥ 130 ॥

130. In such a situation (i.e. during the flow of sushumna)
people desirous of victory, gain and pleasure should
concentrate on the Lord of the Universe and should
indulge in yogic practices only and nothing else.

सूर्येण वहमानायां सुषुम्नायां मुहुर्मुहुः ।
शापंदद्याद्वरं दद्यात्सर्वथैव तदन्यथा ॥ 131 ॥

131. If sushumna flows again and again during the reign of
surya nadi (pingala), then whether you curse or bless,
both are ineffective.

नाडीसंक्रमणे काले तत्त्वसङ्गमनेऽपि च ।
शुभं किञ्चिन्न कर्तव्यं पुण्यदानादि किञ्चन ॥ 132 ॥

132. During the changeover of swara or when the tattwas combine, no auspicious work like acquiring virtues or giving donations, etc. should be done.

विषमस्योदयो यत्र मनसाऽपि न चिन्तयेत् ।
यात्रा हानिकरी तस्य मृत्यु: क्लेशो न संशय: ॥ 133 ॥

133. When the uneven (irregular) swara flows, one should not even think about travelling. It indicates there will be trouble on the journey, harm and sometimes death occurs, there is no doubt.

पुरो वामोर्ध्वतश्चन्द्रोदक्षाध: पृष्ठतो रवि: ।
पूर्णारिक्ताविवेकोऽयं ज्ञातव्यो देशिकै: सदा ॥ 134 ॥

134. If the breath flows from front, left or upper sides in the lunar swara and from right, bottom or back sides in the solar swara, then these should be considered as flowing full strength, otherwise they are empty. This knowledge of discrimination between full and empty swara should always be possessed by the spiritual teachers.

ऊर्ध्ववामाग्रतो दूतो ज्ञेयो वामपथि स्थित: ।
पृष्ठे दक्षे तथाऽधस्तात्सूर्यवाहागत: शुभ: ॥ 135 ॥

135. It is auspicious if the messenger arrives from higher, left or front sides while the lunar swara is flowing, or if he comes from the back, right or lower sides when the solar swara is flowing.

अनादिर्विषम: सन्धिर्निराहारो निराकुल: ।
परे सूक्ष्मे विलीयेत सा सन्ध्या सद्भिरुच्यते ॥ 136 ॥

136. If during the flow of a beginningless irregular sushumna, one, remaining without food and fully engrossed, obtains absorption in the subtle Brahman, then such a sushumna is called sandhya (meeting point) by the knowers.

न वेदं वेद इत्याहुर्वेदो वेदो न विद्यते ।
परात्मा वेद्यते येन स वेदो वेद उच्चते ॥ 137 ॥

137. Mere intellectual knowledge is not considered as Veda and in fact the Vedas are not mere knowing. Veda is said to be that from which knowledge of the supreme spirit is obtained.

न सन्ध्या सन्धिरित्याहुः सन्ध्या सन्धिर्निगद्यते ।
विषमः सन्धिगः प्राणः स सन्धिः सन्धिरुच्यते ॥ 138 ॥

138. Sandhya is not sandhi (the meeting of day and night); this is the external process only. The real sandhi is when the irregular pranas start to flow in sushumna. That is the true sandhi.

श्री देव्युवाच
देवदेव   महादेव   सर्वसंसारतारक ।
स्थितं त्वदीयहृदयेयद्रहस्यं वद मे प्रभो ॥ 139 ॥

139. Devi said:
Deva, Deva, Mahadeva, O saviour of the entire universe, tell me more about this secret knowledge you keep in your heart.

ईश्वर उवाच
स्वरज्ञानरहस्यातु न काचिच्चेष्टदेवता ।
स्वरज्ञानरतोयोगी स योगी परमो मतः ॥ 140 ॥

152

140. Ishwara said:
There is no ishta devata (desired deity) beyond the mystery of the knowledge of swara. A yogi who is engaged in acquisition of the knowledge of swara is considered to be the supreme yogi.

पञ्चतत्त्वाद्भवेत्सृष्टिस्तत्त्वे तत्त्वं प्रलीयते ।
पञ्चतत्त्वं परं तत्त्वं तत्त्वातीतो निरञ्जनः ॥ 141 ॥

141. Creation manifests from the five elements and merges back into them. The five elements are the supreme elements and the supreme Brahma alone is beyond them.

तत्त्वानां नाम विज्ञेयं सिद्धियोगेन योगिभिः ।
भूतानां दुष्टचिह्नानि जानातीह स्वरोत्तमः ॥ 142 ॥

142. Through the means of their siddhis the yogis should know the names of the elements. A person having expertise in swara yoga can recognize the evil qualities of all types of creatures.

पृथिव्यापस्तथा तेजो वायुराकाशमेव च ।
पञ्चभूतात्मकं विश्वं यो जानाति स पूजितः ॥ 143 ॥

143. The person who realizes the universe as being a combination of these five elements (i.e. earth, water, fire, air and ether) is the one to be revered.

सर्वलोकस्थजीवानां न देहो भिन्नतत्त्वकः ।
भूलोकात्सत्यपर्यन्तं नाडीभेदः पृथक्पृथक् ॥ 144 ॥

144. The bodies of the living beings residing in all the lokas from earth to satyaloka are made up of the same elements (tattwas) without exception, but the nadis are different in different bodies.

वामे वा दक्षिणे वाऽपि उदया: पञ्च कीर्तिता: ।
अष्टधा तत्त्वविज्ञानं शृणु वक्ष्यामि सुन्दरि ॥ 145 ॥

145. Five risings have been described in both the left and right sides. O beautiful Parvati, now listen as I explain the eightfold science of the tattwas.

प्रथमे तत्त्वसंख्यानं द्वितीये श्वाससन्धय: ।
तृतीये स्वरचिह्नानि चतुर्थे स्थानमेव च ॥ 146 ॥

146. In the first division is the number of elements; in the second division is the junction of the swara; third is the sign of the swara, and fourth is the place of the swara.

पञ्चमे तस्य वर्णाश्च षष्ठे तु प्राण एव च ।
सप्तमे स्वादसंयुक्ता अष्टमे गतिलक्षणम् ॥ 147 ॥

147. The fifth division is the colour; sixth is the prana; seventh is the taste; eighth is the indication of movement.

एवमष्टविधं प्राणं विषुवन्तं चराचरम् ।
स्वरात्परतरं देवि नान्यथा त्वम्बुजेक्षणे ॥ 148 ॥

148. In this manner, eight categories of prana pervade the entire animate and inanimate creation. O lotus-eyed goddess, there is no knowledge so precious as the wisdom of swara.

निरीक्षितव्यं यत्नेन सदा प्रत्यूषकालत: ।
कालस्य वञ्चनार्थाय कर्मकुर्वन्ति योगिन: ॥ 149 ॥

149. The swara should always be watched carefully from early morning, for it is the means deployed by yogis for escaping from the 'grip' of time.

DESCRIPTION OF SHANMUKHI MUDRA

श्रुत्योरंगुष्ठौ मध्यांगुल्यौ नासापुट्द ये ।
वदनप्रान्तके चान्यांगुलीर्दद्याच्च नेत्रयोः ॥ १५० ॥

150. Fix the thumbs in the ears, close the two nostrils with
the middle fingers, the mouth with the ring and little
fingers and the eyes with the forefingers.

अस्यान्तस्तु पृथिव्यादि तत्त्वज्ञानं भवेत्क्रमात् ।
पीतश्वेतारुणश्यामैर्बिन्दुभिर्निरुपाधिकम्   ॥ १५१ ॥

151. After doing this, knowledge of the elements like earth,
etc. comes serially with careful observation in the form
of yellow, white, red, black and dots of all colours.

दर्पणेन समालोक्य तत्र विनिःक्षिपेत् ।
आकारैस्तु विजानीयात्तत्त्वभेदं विचक्षणः ॥ १५२ ॥

152. Looking into a mirror, one should breathe on it. A
clear-sighted wise person can have knowledge of the
different tattwas on the basis of the shape formed on
the mirror.

चतुरस्रं चार्धचन्द्रं त्रिकोणं वर्तुलं स्मृतम् ।
बिन्दुभिस्तु नभो ज्ञेयमाकारैस्तत्त्वलक्षणम् ॥ १५३ ॥

153. The shapes are known to be a square or quadrangle, a
half-moon, a triangle, a circle, and if it is formed of small
dots, it indicates the presence of the akasha element.

मध्ये पृथ्वी ह्यधश्चापश्चोर्ध्वं वहति चानलः ।
तियेग्वायुप्रवाहश्च नभो वहति संक्रमे ॥ १५४ ॥

154. Earth flows in the middle, water flows downward, fire
flows upward, and air flows at an angle. When the swaras
flow together, know that the ether element is active.

155

COLOUR

आप: श्वेता: क्षिति: पीता रक्तवर्णो हुताशन: ।
मारुतो नीलजीमूत आकाश: सर्ववर्णक: ॥ 155 ॥

155. Water is white; earth is yellow; fire is red; air is cloud-
blue; ether is of mixed colours.

LOCATION OF THE TATTWAS

स्कन्धद्वये स्थितो वह्निर्नाभिमूले प्रभञ्जन: ।
जानुदेशे क्षितिस्तोयं पादान्ते मस्तके नभ: ॥ 156 ॥

156. Fire is located in both the shoulders, air at the root of
the navel, earth in the region of the knees, water in the
feet and ether in the forehead.

TASTE

माहेयं मधुरं स्वादे कषायं जलमेव च ।
तीक्ष्णं तेज: समीरोऽम्ल: आकाशं कटुकं तथा ॥ 157 ॥

157. In taste, earth is sweet, water is astringent, fire is
pungent, air is sour and ether is bitter.

MOTION

अष्टाङ्गुलं वहेद्वायुरनलश्चचतुरङ्गुलम् ।
द्वादशाङ्गुल माहेयं वारुणं षोडशाङ्गुलम् ॥ 158 ॥

158. The length of the swara of the air element is eight
angulas (finger's breadth); of the fire element four
angulas; of the earth element twelve angulas, and of the
water element sixteen angulas.

ऊर्ध्वं मृत्युरध: शान्तिस्तिर्यगुच्चाटनं तथा ।
मध्ये स्तम्भं विजानीयान्नभ: सर्वत्र मध्यमम् ॥ 159 ॥

159. If the swara flows in an upward direction, it indicates death. A downward flow indicates tranquillity. If it flows in an oblique manner, it is a good time for getting rid of bad elements. The flow in the middle indicates motionlessness. The effect of akasha element is moderate in all kinds of works.

पृथिव्यां स्थिरकर्माणि चरकर्माणि वारुणे ।
तेजसि क्रूरकर्माणि मारणोच्चाटनेऽनिले ॥ १६० ॥

160. During the predominance of the earth element it is the time for steady actions; during water for moving work; during fire for difficult actions; during air for actions harmful to others.

व्योम्नि किञ्चिन्न कर्तव्यमभ्यसेद्योगसेवनम् ।
शून्यता सर्वकार्येषु नात्रकार्या विचारणा ॥ १६१ ॥

161. No work should be done at the time of the predominance of the ether element as everything draws a blank during this period. However, yoga sadhana should be done without any other consideration during such a period.

पृथ्वीजलाभ्यांसिद्धिः स्यान्मृत्युर्वह्नौ क्षयोऽनिले ।
नभसो निष्फलं सर्वं ज्ञातव्यं तत्त्ववादिभिः ॥ १६२ ॥

162. Earth and water bring accomplishment, fire brings death, air brings destruction, but ether brings no result. This should be known to the tattwavadis (those who study the elements).

चिरलाभः क्षितौज्ञेयस्तत्क्षणे तोयतत्त्वतः ।
हानिः स्याद्वह्निवाताभ्यां नभसोनिष्फलं भवेत् ॥ १६३ ॥

163. When earth flows, it brings permanent benefits, water brings immediate success, fire and air result in harm and loss, ether bears no fruit.

पीत: शनैर्मध्यवाही हनुर्यावद्गुरुध्वनि: ।
कवोष्ण: पार्थिवो वायु: स्थिरकार्यप्रसाधक: ॥ 164 ॥

164. Indications of the predominance of the earth element in the swara are its yellow colour, slow speed, reaching down to the chin with a heavy sound and slight warmth. This provides success in all kinds of steady works.

अधोवाही गुरुध्वान: शीघ्रग: शीतल: स्थित: ।
य: षोडशाङ्गुलोवायु: स आप: शुभकर्मकृत् ॥ 165 ॥

165. The water element predominant swara flows down-wards, is heavy sounding, flows with fast speed, is cool and extends up to sixteen angulas (in breadth). This is suitable for performing auspicious activities.

आवर्त्तगश्चात्युष्णश्च शोणाभश्चतुरङ्गुल: ।
ऊर्ध्ववाही च य: क्रूरकर्मकारी स तैजस: ॥ 166 ॥

166. The fire element predominant swara flows in a circular motion, is very hot, is blood-red in colour, extends up to four fingers in length, flows upwards and is only suitable for performing cruel actions.

उष्ण: शीत: कृष्णवर्णस्तिर्यग्गाम्यष्टकाङ्गुल: ।
वायु: पवनसंज्ञस्तु चरकर्मप्रसाधक: ॥ 167 ॥

167. The air element predominant swara is temperate, black (or dark) coloured, flows in an oblique direction and extends up to eight (angulas) fingers in breadth. Its name is pavana and it brings about success in dynamic actions.

य: समीर: समरस: सर्वतत्त्वगुणावह: ।
अम्बरंतंविजानीयाद्योगिनां योगदायकम् ॥ 168 ॥

168. The swara which carries the qualities of all the other elements in a balanced manner should be known as (predominated by) ambara, (i.e. ether). This provides success to yogis in learning yoga.

पीतवर्णं चतुष्कोणं मधुरं मध्यमाश्रितम् ।
भोगदं पार्थिवं तत्त्वं प्रवाहे द्वादशाङ्गुलम् ॥ 169 ॥

169. The earth element predominated swara is yellow in colour, quadrangular in shape, sweet in taste and flows in the middle, extending up to twelve fingers in breadth, and provides enjoyment.

श्वेतमर्धेन्दुसंकाशं स्वादुकाषायमार्द्रकम् ।
लाभकृद्द्वारुणं तत्त्वं प्रवाहे षोडशाङ्गुलम् ॥ 170 ॥

170. The water element predominated swara is white in colour, shaped like a half-moon, astringent in taste, damp, and its flow extends up to sixteen angulas in breadth. This bestows all profit and gain.

रक्तं त्रिकोणं तीक्ष्णं च ऊर्ध्वभागप्रवाहकम् ।
दीप्तं च तैजसं तत्त्वं प्रवाहे चतुरङ्गुलम् ॥ 171 ॥

171. The fire element predominated swara is red in colour, triangular in shape, pungent in taste, upward flowing, effulgent, and its flow extends up to four angulas in breadth.

नीलं च वर्तुलाकारं स्वाद्म्लं तिर्यगाश्रितम् ।
चपलं मारुतं तत्त्वं प्रवाहेऽष्टाङ्गुलं स्मृतम् ॥ 172 ॥

172. The air element predominated swara is blue in colour, circular in shape, pleasant-sour in taste, flows at a slant in a fluctuating manner and is said to extend up to eight fingers in breadth.

वर्णाकारे स्वादवाहे अव्यक्तं सर्वगामिनम् ।
मोक्षदं नाभसं तत्त्वं सर्वकार्येषु निष्फलम् ॥ 173 ॥

173. The ether element predominated swara is indistinguishable in colour, shape, taste and flow. It is also all-pervading and provides liberation. However, in all other affairs it is useless.

पृथ्वीजले शुभे तत्त्वे तेजो मिश्रफलोदयम् ।
हानिमृत्युकरौ पुंसामशुभौ व्योममारुतौ ॥ 174 ॥

174. The earth and water elements are auspicious, the fire element gives mixed results, and the ether and air elements are inauspicious and cause loss and death to humans.

आपूर्वपश्चिमे पृथ्वी तेजश्च दक्षिणे तथा ।
वायुश्चोत्तरदिग्ज्ञेयो मध्ये कोणगतं नभः ॥ 175 ॥

175. The earth element extends from east to west, the fire is in the south, the air element should be known to be in the north direction and the ether element resides in the centre in an oblique position.

चन्द्रे पृथ्वीजले स्यातां सूर्येऽग्निर्वा यदा भवेत् ।
तदा सिद्धिर्नसंदेहः सौम्यासौम्येषु कर्मसु ॥ 176 ॥

176. When there is a predominance of the earth or water element in the lunar swara, or there is fire element in the solar swara, then there will be success in all types

of work whether placid or dynamic. There is no doubt about it.

लाभः पृथ्वीकृतोऽह्निः स्यान्निशायां लाभकृज्जलम् ।
वह्नौ मृत्युः क्षयो वायुर्नभस्थानंदहेत्क्वचित् ॥ 177 ॥

177. When the earth element flows during the day or the water element during the night, one obtains profit. Fire brings death, air destruction and ether in some cases causes loss due to fire.

जीवितव्ये जये लाभे कृष्यां च धनकर्मणि ।
मन्त्रार्थे युद्धप्रश्ने च गमनागमने तथा ॥ 178 ॥

178. The elements should be consulted in questions concerning life, victory, profit, farming, money matters (earning), consultations (mantra), and questions related to battle (fighting) and travel.

आयाति वारुणे तत्त्वे शत्रुरस्ति शुभः क्षितौ ।
प्रयाति वायुतोऽन्यत्र हानिमृत्यु नभोऽनले ॥ 179 ॥

179. During the water element the enemy will come; during earth there will be happiness; during air the enemy will go away; during fire and ether there will be harm and death.

TYPES OF THOUGHT

पृथिव्यां मूलचिन्ता स्याज्जीवस्य जलवातयोः ।
तेजसा धातुचिन्तास्याच्छून्यमाकाशतोवदेत् ॥ 180 ॥

180. During the earth element, the mind is orientated towards material thoughts. During water and air, thoughts relate to one's life. In fire, thoughts are about treasure, wealth, etc. In ether, there is no thought or worry, only shoonyata (void).

WALKING

पृथिव्यां बहुपादाः स्यूर्द्विपदस्तोयवायुतः ।
तेजस्येव चतुष्पादो नभसा पादवर्जितः ॥ 181 ॥

181. During the earth element take many steps; during water and air two steps; during fire four steps; during ether don't walk anywhere.

कुजो वह्निः रविः पृथ्वी सौरिरपि: प्रकीर्तित: ।
वायुस्थानस्थितो   राहुर्दक्षरन्ध्रप्रवाहकः ॥ 182 ॥

182. In the right swara, Mars resides in the fire element, the sun in the earth element, Saturn in the water element and Neptune in the air element.

जलं चन्द्रो बुधः पृथ्वी गुरुर्वातः सितोऽनलः ।
वामनाड्यां स्थितः सर्वे सर्वकार्येषु निश्चिताः ॥ 183 ॥

183. In the left swara, the moon resides in the water element, Mercury in the earth element, Jupiter in the air element and Venus in the fire element. All these are definitely auspicious for all types of work.

पृथ्वी बुधो जलादिन्दुः शुक्रो वह्निः रविः कुजः ।
वायु राहुशानी व्योम गुरुरेवं प्रकीर्तितः ॥ 184 ॥

184. Earth signifies Mercury; water the moon and Venus; fire the sun and Mars; air Neptune and Saturn; and ether Jupiter.

QUESTIONS ACCORDING TO THE DIFFERENT DIRECTIONS

प्रवासप्रश्न आदित्ये यदि राहुर्गतोऽनिले ।
तदासौ चलितो ज्ञेयः स्थानान्तरमपेक्षते ॥ 185 ॥

162

185. When a person has gone away and somebody else asks about him, if the questioner is on the side of your active solar swara and Neptune is in the air element, it means that the person is on the move, shifting to another place.

आयाति वारुणे तत्त्वे तत्रैवास्ति शुभः क्षितौ ।
प्रवासी पवनेऽन्यत्र मृत्युरेवानले भवेत् ॥ 186 ॥

186. If the question is asked during the dominance of water element, it means that the person will return. During the earth element it means that he is well and is at the same place. Air means that he has left that place and has gone somewhere else, and fire means that he is no more alive.

DESIRED QUESTIONS

पार्थिवे मूलविज्ञानं शुभं कार्यं जले तथा ।
आग्नेयेधातुविज्ञानं व्योम्नि शून्यंविर्निदशेत् ॥ 187 ॥

187. In the earth element mundane affairs are prosperous, water is good for auspicious work, fire is good for dealing with metals, and in ether there are no concerns or worries.

तुष्टिः पुष्टिः रतिः क्रीडा जयहर्षौ धराजले ।
तेजवाय्वोश्च सुप्ताक्षो ज्वरकम्पः प्रवासिनः ॥ 188 ॥

188. If there is either the earth or water element at the time of a question about someone who has gone out, then the person in question is enjoying a satisfied life, good health, the love of others, entertainment, victory and pleasure. If there is the fire or wind element, then the person is suffering from fever with shivering or excessive sleep.

गतायुर्मृत्युराकाशे तत्त्वस्थाने प्रकीर्तितः ।
द्वादशैता: प्रयत्नेन ज्ञातव्या देशिकै: सदा ॥ 189 ॥

189. If the question is asked during the ether element, the
person is at the end of his life or has already died.
Thus, from the prevailing element during the time
when these twelve types of questions are asked, the
practitioner of tattwa sadhana should know the results.

पूर्वस्यां पश्चिमे याम्ये उत्तरस्यां यथाक्रमम् ।
पृथिव्यादीनि भूतानि बलिष्ठानि विनिर्दिशेत् ॥ 190 ॥

190. The earth, water, fire and air elements are powerful in
the east, west, south and north directions respectively.

पृथिव्यापस्तथा तेजो वायुराकाशमेव च ।
पञ्चभूतात्मको देहो ज्ञातव्यश्च वरानने ॥ 191 ॥

191. O beautiful-faced Parvati, it should be known that
this body is nothing but the combination of the five
elements (i.e. earth, water, fire, air and ether).

PLACE OF THE FIVE ELEMENTS IN THE BODY

अस्थि मांसं त्वचा नाडी रोमं चैव तु पञ्चमम् ।
पृथ्वी पञ्चगुणा प्रोक्ता ब्रह्मज्ञानेन भाषितम् ॥ 192 ॥

192. There are five qualities of the earth element in this
body in the form of bone, flesh, skin, nadis and hair.
This has been said on the strength of Brahma jnana.

शुक्रशोणितमज्जा च मूत्रं लाला च पञ्चमम् ।
आप: पञ्चगुणा: प्रोक्ता: ब्रह्मज्ञानेन भाषितम् ॥ 193 ॥

193. Semen/ova, blood, marrow, urine and saliva are the five
qualities of the water element. This is also told by the
Brahma jnanis.

क्षुधा तृषा तथा निद्रा कान्तिरालस्यमेव च ।
तेज: पञ्चगुणंप्रोक्तं ब्रह्मज्ञानेन भाषितम् ॥ 194 ॥

194. Hunger, thirst, sleep, lustre of body and laziness are the five qualities of the fire element. This is said by the Brahma jnanis.

धावनं चलनं ग्रन्थ: सङ्कोचनप्रसारणे ।
वायो: पञ्चगुणा: प्रोक्ता: ब्रह्मज्ञानेन भाषितम् ॥ 195 ॥

195. Running, walking, glandular secretion, contraction and expansion of the body are the five qualities of the air element. This the Brahma jnanis have said.

रागद्वेषौ तथा लज्जा भयं मोहश्च पञ्चम: ।
नभ: पञ्चगुणं प्रोक्तं ब्रह्मज्ञानेन भाषितम् ॥ 196 ॥

196. Attachment, jealousy, shyness, fear and passion are the five qualities belonging to the ether element. This is said by the Brahma jnanis.

QUESTIONS REGARDING GAIN

पृथिव्या: पलानि पञ्चाशच्चत्वारिंशत्तथाम्भस: ।
अग्नेस्त्रिंशत्पुनर्वायोर्विंशतिर्नभसो   दश ॥ 197 ॥

197. In the body the earth element is 50 palas (parts), water is 40 palas, fire is 30 palas, air 20 palas and ether 10 palas.

पृथिव्यां चिरकालेन लाभश्चाप: क्षणाद्भवेत् ।
जायते पवने स्वल्प: सिद्धोऽप्यग्नौ विनश्यति ॥ 198 ॥

198. The activity of earth ensures long-term success; water gives instant results; in air success is rare; but in fire even an accomplished work will be spoiled.

पृथिव्याः पञ्च ह्यापां वेदा गुणास्तेजो द्विवायुतः ।
नभस्येकगुणश्चैव   तत्त्वज्ञानमिदं   भवेत् ॥ 199 ॥

199. Earth has five qualities, water four, fire three, air two
and ether one. This is the eternal knowledge and these
are the proportions of the elements.

THE PLANET EARTH

फूत्कारकृत्प्रस्फुटिता विदीर्णा पतिता धरा ।
ददाति सर्वकार्येषु अवस्थासदृशं फलम् ॥ 200 ॥

200. The different forms of the swara which is dominated
by the earth element, e.g. producing a hissing sound,
broken (non-continuous), torn (with split sound) and
with downward direction, provides results in all the
works according to its situation (condition).

STAR CONSTELLATIONS AND THE TATTWAS

धनिष्ठा रोहिणी ज्येष्ठाऽनुराधा श्रवणं तथा ।
अभिजिदुत्तराषाढा   पृथ्वीतत्त्वमुदाहृतम् ॥ 201 ॥

201. The earth element is concerned with the stars and
constellations (nakshatras) of: Dhanishta (Delphini),
Rohini (Aldebaran), Jyeshtha (Antares), Anuradha
(Scorpionis), Shravana (Aquitae), Abhijit (Vega) and
Uttarashadha (Sagittari).

पूर्वाषाढा तथाऽऽश्लेषा मूलमार्द्रा च रेवती ।
उत्तराभाद्रपदा तोयतत्त्वं शतभिषक् प्रिये ॥ 202 ॥

202. O dear one, the water element is concerned with the
stars and constellations of: Poorvashadha (Sagittari),
Aslesha (Hydarae), Moola (Scorpionis), Ardra
(Betelguese), Revati (Piscum), Uttarabhadrapada
(Andromedae) and Shatabhishaj (Aquari).

166

भरणी कृत्तिका पुष्यो मघा पूर्वा च फाल्गुनी ।
पूर्वाभाद्रपदा स्वाती तेजस्तत्त्वमिति प्रिये ॥ 203 ॥

203. O beloved one, the stars and constellations concerned
with the fire element are: Bharani (Arietis), Krittika
(Tauri), Pushya (Cancri), Magha (Regulas), Poorva-
phalguni (Leonis), Poorvabhadrapada (Pegasi) and
Swati (Bootis).

विशाखोत्तरफाल्गुन्यौ हस्तचित्रे पुनर्वसुः ।
अश्विनीमृगशीर्षे च वायुतत्त्वमुदाहृतम् ॥ 204 ॥

204. The stars and constellations concerned with the
air element are: Vishakha (Librae), Uttaraphalguni
(Lionis), Hasta (Corvi), Chitra (Virginis), Punarvasu
(Geminorium), Ashwini (Castor and Pollux) and
Mrigashirsha (Orionis).

QUESTIONS OF THE MESSENGER

वहन्नाडीस्थितो दूतो यत्पृच्छति शुभाशुभम् ।
तत्सर्वं सिद्धिमाप्नोति शून्ये शून्यं न संशयः ॥ 205 ॥

205. If a messenger sits or stands on the side of the active
swara and asks either auspicious or inauspicious
questions, all of them will have a positive and successful
outcome. But if he sits on the side of the blocked nadi,
there will be no result, that is certain.

पूर्णेऽपि निर्गमश्वासे सुतत्त्वेऽपि न सिद्धिदः ।
सूर्यश्चन्द्रोऽथवा नृणां संग्रहे सर्वसिद्धिदः ॥ 206 ॥

206. Even if the outgoing breath is flowing full strength with
the predominance of auspicious elements, through
either the solar or the lunar swara, it does not provide
success, but if there is a conjunction of both, then it
gives all kinds of success.

तत्त्वे रामो जयं प्राप्तः सुतत्त्वे च धनञ्जयः ।
कौरवाः निहताः सर्वे युद्धे तत्त्वविपर्ययात् ॥ 207 ॥

207. During the time of the auspicious elements Sri Rama
was victorious and Arjuna also was victorious, but all the
Kauravas were killed during the war due to the reverse
elements.

जन्मान्तरीय संस्कारात्प्रसादादथवा गुरोः ।
केषाञ्चिज्जायते तत्त्ववासना विमलात्मनाम् ॥ 208 ॥

208. Only those few possessing pure hearts and having good
samskaras from previous incarnations or with the guru's
grace receive this knowledge of the elements.

CHARACTERISTICS OF THE TATTWAS

लंबीजं धरणीं ध्यायेच्चतुरस्रां सुपीतभाम् ।
सुगन्धां स्वर्णवर्णाभां प्राप्नुयाद्देहलाघवम् ॥ 209 ॥

209. *Lam* is the seed mantra of the earth element. One
should concentrate on this element which has a shining
yellow-coloured square, a pleasant smell and a golden
light. By this one can obtain lightness of body.

वं बीजं वारुणं ध्यायेत्तत्त्वमर्धशशिप्रभम् ।
क्षुत्तृष्णादिसहिष्णुत्वं जलमध्ये च मज्जनम् ॥ 210 ॥

210. *Vam* is the bija mantra of the water element. By
concentrating on it and the form of a shining crescent
moon, hunger and thirst can be overcome, and one can
stay for a long time under water. Thus one has power
over water.

रं बीजं अग्निं ध्यायेत्त्रिकोणमरुणप्रभम् ।
बह्वन्नपानभोक्तृत्वमातपाग्निसहिष्णुता ॥ 211 ॥

211. One who concentrates on the bija mantra *Ram* of the fire element situated in a shining red triangle can eat and drink colossal amounts of food, and bear the heat of the sun or fire.

यं बीजं पवनं ध्यायेद्वर्तुलं श्यामलप्रभम् ।
आकाशगमनाद्यं च पक्षिवद्गमनं तथा ॥212॥

212. *Yam*, the bija mantra of the air element, should be meditated upon. It is circular and blue or dark in colour. The person who has power over it can move through the air, fly like a bird (experience levitation).

हं बीजं गगनं ध्यायेन्निराकारं बहुप्रभम् ।
ज्ञानं त्रिकालविषयमैश्वर्यमणिमादिकम् ॥213॥

213. For concentration on the ether element, which is formless and multicoloured, one uses the bija mantra *Ham*. Through these practices comes the knowledge of past, present and future and gain of prosperity, jewels, gems, etc.

THE IMPORTANT POINT OF SWARA YOGA

स्वरज्ञानी नरो यत्र धनं नास्ति ततः परम् ।
गम्यते स्वरज्ञानेन ह्यनायासं फलं भवेत् ॥214॥

214. There is no wealth greater than the wisdom of the practitioner of the swara science, because the person who acts according to the swara gains results without effort.

श्रीदेव्युवाच
देवदेव महादेव महाज्ञानं स्वरोदयम् ।
त्रिकालविषयं चैव कथं भवति शंकर ॥215॥

215. Devi said:

O God of gods, Mahadeva, how does this great science of swarodaya provide knowledge of past, present and future?

ईश्वर उवाच
अर्थकालजयप्रश्न शुभाशुभमिति त्रिधा ।
एतत्त्रिकालविज्ञानं नान्यद्भवति सुन्दरि ॥216॥

216. Ishwara said:

O beautiful one, there are three types of auspicious or inauspicious questions pertaining to wealth, kala (i.e. time related to life) and victory belonging to past, present and future. This knowledge of past, present and future can be had only through swara yoga and nothing else.

तत्त्वे शुभाशुभं कार्यं तत्त्वे जयपराजयौ ।
तत्त्वे सुभिक्षदुर्भिक्षे तत्त्वं त्रिपदमुच्यते ॥217॥

217. By the tattwa only, one can distinguish auspicious/inauspicious events, victory/defeat, abundance of food or famine. Thus the tattwas are said to be the cause of the works of all three times.

श्रीदेव्युवाच
देवदेव   महादेव   सर्वसंसारसागरे ।
किं नराणां परं मित्रं सर्वकार्यार्थसाधकम् ॥218॥

218. Devi said:

Deva, Deva, Mahadeva, O God of all gods, in this universe who is the greatest friend of humans and what is that by which all desires can be fulfilled?

ईश्वर उवाच
प्राण एव परं मित्रं प्राण एव पर: सखा ।
प्राणतुल्य: परो बन्धुर्नास्ति नास्ति वरानने ॥219॥

170

219. Ishwara said:
Prana is the greatest friend, prana is the greatest companion. O fair-faced one there is no closer friend in this universe than prana.

श्रीदेव्युवाच
कथं प्राणस्थितो वायुर्देह: किं प्राणरूपक: ।
तत्त्वेषु संचरन्प्राणो ज्ञायते योगिभि: कथम् ॥ 220 ॥

220. Devi said:
How does the air reside in the prana, and is the body in the form of prana? How is the prana moving in the tattwas perceived by the yogis?

शिव उवाच
कायानगरमध्यस्थो मारुतो रक्षपालक: ।
प्रवेशे दशभि: प्रोक्तो निर्गमे द्वादशांगुल: ॥ 221 ॥

221. Shiva said:
Residing in the centre of this body, prana vayu is like a guard. On entering the body (inhalation) it is said to be ten fingers long, on leaving (exhalation) it is twelve.

गमने तु चतुर्विंशन्नेत्रवेदास्तु धावने ।
मैथुने पञ्चषष्टिश्च शयने च शतांगुलम् ॥ 222 ॥

222. At the time of walking it is twenty-four fingers; running, forty-two; copulating, sixty-five; sleeping, one hundred.

प्राणस्य तु गतिर्देवि स्वभावाद्द्वादशांगुला ।
भोजने वमने चैव गतिरष्टादशांगुला ॥ 223 ॥

223. O Devi, prana is naturally twelve fingers in length, but while eating or vomiting it is eighteen.

एकाङ्गुले कृते न्यूने प्राणे निष्कामता मता ।
आनन्दस्तु द्वितीये स्यात्कामशक्तिस्तृतीयके ॥224॥

224. If a yogi succeeds in reducing the length of prana by
one finger (out of twelve fingers), he obtains desire-
lessness, with a reduction of two fingers he gets bliss,
if reduced by three fingers he gets the energy of love
(sex).

वाचासिद्धिश्चतुर्थे च दूरदृष्टिस्तु पञ्चमे ।
षष्ठे त्वाकाशगमनं चण्डवेगश्च सप्तमे ॥225॥

225. Reduction of the length of prana by four fingers gives
the power of speech (whatever one says comes true);
five, telepathy; six, the ability to levitate; seven enables
one to move with enormous speed.

अष्टमे सिद्धयश्चैव नवमे निधयो नव ।
दशमे दशमूर्तिश्च छाया नैकादशे भवेत् ॥226॥

226. Reduction of the length of prana by eight fingers gives
attainment of the eight siddhis (perfections); nine,
attainment of the nine nidhis (riches); ten, ability to
change the body into ten forms; eleven, the ability to
make the body shadowless.

द्वादशे हंसचारश्च गङ्गाऽमृतरसं पिबेत् ।
आनखाग्रं प्राणपूर्णे कस्य भक्ष्यं च भोजनम् ॥227॥

227. Reduction of the length of prana by twelve fingers
enables one to attain the state of hamsa and drink the
nectar of the Ganga (to become immortal). The yogi who
achieves control over the prana, right from his toes to
his head, needs no food and has no desire to eat.

एवं प्राणविधिः प्रोक्तः सर्वकार्यफलप्रदः ।
ज्ञायते गुरुवाक्येन न विद्याशास्त्रकोटिभिः ॥228॥

228. Thus the method of achieving all kinds of success through control of prana has been described. This knowledge comes only through the guru's instruction, and no amount of study can provide it.

प्रातश्चन्द्रो रवि: सायं यदि दैवान्न लभ्यते ।
मध्याह्नमध्यरात्र्याश्च परतस्तु प्रवर्तते ॥ 229 ॥

229. If by chance the lunar swara does not flow in the morning, or the solar in the evening, they will come in force after midday or midnight.

QUESTIONS ON WAR

दूरयुद्धे जयी चन्द्र: समासन्ने दिवाकर: ।
वह्नाङ्यागत: पाद: सर्वसिद्धिप्रदायक: ॥ 230 ॥

230. If one wants to fight in a distant country, one should follow chandra swara for victory. If one has to go to battle in a nearby country, one should start in pingala. Step forward with the same foot as the active swara and it will provide all kinds of success.

यात्रारम्भे विवाहे च प्रवेशे नगरादिके ।
शुभकार्याणि सिद्धयन्ति चन्द्रचारेषु सर्वदा ॥ 231 ॥

231. At the start of a journey, at the time of marriage or while entering into a city, and for all auspicious works the lunar swara should be active in order to get success.

अयनतिथिदिनेशै: स्वीयतत्त्वे च युक्ते ।
यदिवहति कदाचिद्दैवयोगेन पुंसाम् ।
स जयति रिपुसैन्यं स्तम्भमात्रस्वरेण
प्रभवति न च विघ्नं केशवस्यापि लोके ॥ 232 ॥

232. If by good fortune the presiding deities of the northern and southern course of the sun, the lunar day and

the solar day are present with their elements in one's breath, one can conquer the enemy army merely by holding one's breath, and there will be no obstacle in the spiritual world of Lord Keshava.

जीवं रक्ष जीवं रक्ष जीवाङ्गे परिधाय च ।
जीवो जपति यो युद्धे जीवञ्जयति मेदिनीम् ॥ 233 ॥

233. One who covers his chest with his cloth and repeatedly utters the mantra *Jivam raksha* (save my soul) during battle, survives and also conquers the whole earth.

भूमौ जले च कर्तव्यं गमनं शान्तिकर्मसु ।
वह्नौ वायौ प्रदीप्तेषु खे पुनर्नोभयेष्वपि ॥ 234 ॥

234. It is appropriate to travel for peaceful purposes during the flow of the earth or water element, for difficult and dynamic actions during the flow of the air or fire element, and for neither of the two during the flow of the ether element.

जीवेन शस्त्रं बध्नीयाज्जीवेनैव विकासयेत् ।
जीवेन प्रक्षिपेच्छस्त्रं युद्धे जयति सर्वदा ॥ 235 ॥

235. The person who holds a weapon in the same hand as the active swara, who uses it with the same hand, aims and throws it with the same hand, always wins the battle.

आकृष्य प्राणपवनं समारोहेत वाहनम् ।
समुत्तरे पदं दद्यात्सर्वकार्याणि साधयेत् ॥ 236 ॥

236. One who draws in the prana vayu while mounting any vehicle and who puts his foot on the upper part of it obtains success in all affairs.

अपूर्णे शत्रुसामग्रीं पूर्णे वा स्वबलं तथा ।
कुरुते पूर्णतत्त्वस्थो जयत्येको वसुन्धराम् ॥ 237 ॥

237. Flowing under the full influence of the appropriate
element, an empty swara provides the advantage
in war materials to the enemy, but when flowing
full strength, it increases one's fighting power to
the extent that one could conquer the earth single-
handed.

या नाडी वहते चाङ्गे तस्यामेवाधिदेवता ।
सम्मुखेऽपदिशा तेषां सर्वकार्यफलप्रदा ॥ 238 ॥

238. When the swara flows with the appropriate nadi and
the presiding deity and the proper direction are on the
same side, all desires are fulfilled.

आदौ तु क्रियते मुद्रा पश्चाद्युद्धं समाचरेत् ।
सर्पमुद्रा कृता येन तस्य सिद्धिर्नसंशयः ॥ 239 ॥

239. One should initially practise mudra and then start
fighting. The person who does sarpamudra obtains
success without doubt.

चन्द्रप्रवाहेऽप्यथ सूर्यवाहे
भटाः समायान्ति च योद्धुकामाः ।
समीरणस्तत्त्वविदां प्रतीतो
या शून्यता सा प्रतिकार्य नाशिनी ॥ 240 ॥

240. If all brave fighters with the desire to fight go to war
either during the lunar or solar swara when the air
element is in force, then it is auspicious. If the closed
swara is followed instead, destruction ensures.

यां दिशं वहते वायुर्युद्धं तद्दिद्दिशि दापयेत् ।
जयत्येव न सन्देहः शक्रोऽपि यदि चाग्रतः ॥ 241 ॥

241. The battle should be forced to be fought on the side on which one's swara is flowing. Thus one will win without any doubt, even if Indra is opposing one.

यत्र नाड्यां वहेद्वायुस्तदङ्गेप्राणमेव च ।
आकृष्य गच्छेत्कर्णान्तं जयत्येव पुरन्दरम् ॥ 242 ॥

242. One should go (to the battlefield) after drawing the prana up to the ear on the side of the active swara, then one will definitely conquer Indra.

प्रतिपक्षप्रहारेभ्य: पूर्णाङ्गं योभिरक्षति ।
न तस्य रिपुभिर्शक्तिर्बलिष्ठैरपि हन्यते ॥ 243 ॥

243. (During battle) one who protects the side (of the body) corresponding to the active swara, when assaulted by the enemy, becomes so strong that even powerful enemies cannot defeat him.

अंगुष्ठतर्जनीवंशे पादांगुष्ठे तथा ध्वनि: ।
युद्धकाले च कर्तव्यो लक्षयोद्धुजयो भवेत् ॥ 244 ॥

244. During battle one who can make a sound with the thumb and the upper part of the first finger, or from the big toe, can defeat a hundred thousand fighters.

निशाकरे रवौ चारे मध्ये यस्य समीरण: ।
स्थितो रक्षेद्रिद्दगन्तानि जयकांक्षीगत: सदा ॥ 245 ॥

245. One who desires victory and goes to war during the flow of either ida or pingala when the air element is active can protect (his army or country borders) from all directions, even while remaining stationary.

EXAMINING THE MESSENGER

श्वासप्रवेशकाले तु दूतो जल्पति वाञ्छितम् ।
तस्यार्थः सिद्धिमायाति निर्गमे नैव सुन्दरि ॥ 246 ॥

246. If a messenger should speak about a desire at the time
of inhalation, it will be fulfilled, O beautiful one, but at
the time of exhalation it will not.

लाभादीन्यपि कार्याणि पृष्टानि कीर्तितानि च ।
जीवेविशतिसिद्धयन्ति हानिर्निस्सरणे भवेत् ॥ 247 ॥

247. All actions related to gain, etc. questioned or
explained at the time of inhalation are successful.
During exhalation one only gets losses.

नरे दक्षा स्वकीया च स्त्रियां वामा प्रशस्यते ।
कुम्भको युद्धकाले च तिस्रोनाड्यस्त्रयीगतिः ॥ 248 ॥

248. The right swara is auspicious for men and the left is
auspicious for women. At the time of battle no swara
(i.e. kumbhaka) is best. In this manner, there are three
nadis and three directions of flow.

हकारस्य सकारस्य विना भेदं स्वरः कथम् ।
सोऽहं हंसपदेनैव जीवो जयति सर्वदा ॥ 249 ॥

249. How can there be any knowledge of the swara without
knowledge of the syllables *Ha* and *Sa*? Repetition of the
mantra *So-Ham* and *Ham-So* always leads to success.

शून्याङ्गं पूरितं कृत्वा जीवाङ्गे गोपयेज्जयम् ।
जीवाङ्गे घातमाप्नोति शून्याङ्गं रक्षते सदा ॥ 250 ॥

250. By inhaling fully through the closed swara (and
retaining through kumbhaka), one should guard victory
(to come) through the active swara. This strategy is

necessary because affliction comes on the side of the open swara and the closed swara always protects.

वामे वा यदि वा दक्षे यदि पृच्छति पृच्छकः ।
पूर्णे घातो न जायेत शून्ये घातं विनिर्दिशेत् ॥251॥

251. If a messenger asks about war when either the lunar or solar swara is fully flowing, it indicates no loss. But if it is closed, then loss (destruction) is certain.

TYPES OF INJURY

भूतत्त्वेनोदरे घातः पदस्थानेऽम्बुना भवेत् ।
ऊरुस्थानेऽग्नितत्त्वेन करस्थाने च वायुना ॥252॥

252. If the earth element is predominant at the time of a question about war damages, then there will be an injury in the stomach; if the water element predominates, then the legs will be injured; if the fire element predominates, then the thighs will be injured; and if the air element predominates, the hands will be injured.

शिरसि व्योमतत्त्वे च ज्ञातव्यो घातनिर्णयः ।
एवं पञ्चविधो घातः स्वरशास्त्रे प्रकाशितः ॥253॥

253. Similarly, if the ether element is in force, injury comes to the head. In this way, there are five types of injury according to the Swarodaya shastra.

युद्धकाले यदा चन्द्रः स्थायी जयति निश्चितम् ।
यदा सूर्यप्रवाहस्तु यायी विजयते तदा ॥254॥

254. If during battle the lunar swara flows, the ruler of the home country (the invaded) is undoubtedly victorious. If the solar swara flows, then the army of the other country (the invader) is victorious.

178

जयमध्ये तु सन्देहे नाडीमध्यं तु लक्षयेत् ।
सुषुम्नायां गते प्राणे समरे शत्रुसङ्कटम् ॥ २५५ ॥

255. If there is any doubt about victory one should check
the flow of prana in the middle nadi (i.e. sushumna).
If sushumna is flowing, then there is danger from the
enemy in the battle.

यस्यां नाड्यां भवेच्चारस्तां दिशं युधि संश्रयेत् ।
तदाऽसौ जयमाप्नोति नात्रकार्या विचारणा ॥ २५६ ॥

256. If a person takes shelter or makes his base during a
battle in the direction of the active swara, then he gains
victory; there is no need to give it a second thought.

यदि संग्रामकाले तु वामनाडी सदावहेत् ।
स्थायिनो विजयं विद्याद्रिपुवश्यादयोऽपि च ॥ २५७ ॥

257. If the lunar nadi flows continuously at the time of battle,
the invaded side will gain victory and the enemy (the
invader) will also be captured or kept under control.

यदि संग्रामकाले तु सूर्यस्तु व्यावृतो वहेत् ।
तदा यायिजयं विद्यात्सदेवासुरमानवे ॥ २५८ ॥

258. If during battle the flow of the solar swara becomes
non-continuous or ceases, then the invader will gain
victory. This is true for the manavas (humans) as well
as for the devas (gods) and the asuras (demons).

रणे हरति शत्रुस्तं वामायां प्रविशेन्नरः ।
स्थानं विषुवचारेण जयः सूर्येण धावता ॥ २५९ ॥

259. One who enters the war during the flow of his lunar
swara will be captured by the enemy. If he enters during
the flow of sushumna nadi, the enemy will capture his
territory. If he enters during the flow of the solar swara,
then he will gain victory.

179

युद्धद्वये कृते प्रश्ने पूर्णस्य प्रथमे जयः ।
रिक्ते चैवद्वितीयस्तु जयी भवति नान्यथा ॥ 260 ॥

260. If questions are asked about the outcome of two wars
or of two fronts of a war when the swara is fully open,
then there will be victory in the war (or at the war front)
pertaining to the first question. If the swara is closed,
then there will be victory in the war (or at the war front)
pertaining to the second question, not otherwise.

पूर्णनाडीगतः पृष्ठे शून्याङ्गं च तदाग्रतः ।
शून्यस्थाने कृतः शत्रुर्म्रियते नात्र संशयः ॥ 261 ॥

261. If one follows the full swara at the time of going to
war, the enemy will trouble him. If he starts at the time
of the closed swara, he will come face to face with the
enemy. If he keeps the enemy on the side of his closed
swara, then the death of the enemy is certain.

QUESTIONS CONCERNING WAR

वामचारे समं नाम यस्य तस्य जयो भवेत् ।
पृच्छको दक्षिणे भागे विजयी विषमाक्षरः ॥ 262 ॥

262. When the lunar swara is flowing, the person whose
name is simple and common or contains an even
number of letters gains victory. However, if the
questioner is on the right side, then the person whose
name is unusual or has an odd number of letters is
victorious.

यदा पृच्छति चन्द्रस्य तदा सन्धानमादिशेत् ।
पृच्छेद्यदा तु सूर्यस्य तदा जानीहि विग्रहम् ॥ 263 ॥

263. If the lunar swara flows while questioning, then there
will be a compromise. If the solar swara flows, then
know that there will be war.

पार्थिवे च समं युद्धं सिद्धिर्भवति वारुणे ।
युद्धेहि तेजसो भङ्गो मृत्युर्वायौ नभस्यपि ॥ 264 ॥

264. If the question is asked during the dominance of the
earth element, then the results will be equal for both
parties; during the water element, the questioner will
win; during the fire element, the questioner will face
destruction or injury; and during the air and ether
elements, the questioner will die.

निमित्ताद्वाप्रमादाद्वा यदा न ज्ञायतेऽनिल: ।
पृच्छाकाले तदा कुर्यादिदं यत्नेन बुद्धिमान् ॥ 265 ॥

265. If out of carelessness or for any other reason one does
not know which swara is flowing at the time of an
inquiry into the future, an intelligent person should
carefully do the following:

निश्चलां धारणां कृत्वा पुष्पं हस्तान्निपातयेत् ।
पूर्णाङ्गे पुष्पपतनं शून्यं वा तत्परं भवेत् ॥ 266 ॥

266. Holding the mind steady, drop a flower from the hand.
The flower will fall to the side of the flowing swara and
therefore the other side will be the empty one.

तिष्ठन्नुपविशञ्चापि प्राणमाकर्षयन्निजम् ।
मनोभङ्गमकुर्वाण: सर्वकार्येषु जीवति ॥ 267 ॥

267. While standing or sitting, if the person draws in his
prana vayu with full concentration, he will be successful
in every sphere.

न कालो विविधं घोरं न शस्त्रं न च पन्नगा: ।
न शत्रुर्व्याधिचौराद्या: शून्यस्थानाशितुं क्षमा: ॥ 268 ॥

268. When one is merged in the flow of sushumna, then
even the most horrible times (kala), weapons, snakes,

the enemy, disease, a thief, etc. are unable to destroy or cause him suffering.

जीवेन स्थापयेद्वायुं जीवेनारम्भयेत्पुन: ।
जीवेन क्रीडते नित्यं द्यूते जयति सर्वथा ॥ 269 ॥

269. A person who, through the vital prana, establishes the deity presiding over wind and then begins activities regarding playing with dice and takes pleasure in playing, always becomes victorious.

स्वरज्ञानबलादग्रे निष्फलं कोटिधा भवेत् ।
इहलोके परत्रापि स्वरज्ञानी बली सदा ॥ 270 ॥

270. Crores of other kinds of power are useless before the strength of the knowledge of the swara. One who has this knowledge is always powerful both in this world as well as the next.

दशशतायुतं लक्षं देशाधिपबलं क्वचित् ।
शतक्रतुसुरेन्द्राणां बलं कोटिगुणं भवेत् ॥ 271 ॥

271. Some possess the strength of ten people, some of a hundred, some of ten thousand, some of a hundred thousand and some are equal in strength to the king of the country. But the strength of the person who has knowledge of the swara has a crore times the strength of a hundred Indras.

श्री देव्युवाच
परस्परं मनुष्याणां युद्धे प्रोक्तो जयस्त्वया ।
यमयुद्धे समुत्पन्ने मनुष्याणां कथं जय: ॥ 272 ॥

272. Devi said:
You have explained about success in war between human beings. But what if one has to face battle with

182

the lord of death (Yamaraja). How will humans be victorious then?

ईश्वर उवाच
ध्यायेद्देवं स्थिरो जीवं जुहुयाज्जीवसङ्गमे ।
इष्टसिद्धिर्भवेत्तस्य महालाभो जयस्तथा ॥ 273 ॥

273. Ishwara said:
One who meditates upon God with a still and undisturbed mind and who submits the oblation of his vital breath in kumbhaka (i.e. stops his prana vayu) has his desires fulfilled and gains immense benefit and victory.

निराकारात्समुत्पन्नं साकारं सकलं जगत् ।
तत्साकारं निराकारं ज्ञानं भवति तत्क्षणात् ॥ 274 ॥

274. The whole world of forms has originated from the formless God. By the practice of oblation as explained above (in the previous verse), real knowledge of the world of forms and the formless supreme Lord comes instantly.

श्री देव्युवाच
नरयुद्धं च यमयुद्धं त्वयाप्रोक्तं महेश्वर ।
इदानीं देव देवानांवशीकरणकं वद ॥ 275 ॥

275. Devi said:
O Maheshwara! You explained the technique for victory in the fight with men and death (Yamaraja). Now, O God of gods, kindly tell me about the science of captivation.

CAPTIVATING WOMAN

ईश्वर उवाच
चन्द्रं सूर्येण चाकृष्य स्थापयेज्जीवमण्डले ।
आजन्मवशगा रामा कथितोऽयं तपोधनै: ॥ 276 ॥

276. Ishwara said:
If the (woman's) lunar swara is taken through the (man's) solar swara and he retains it in his jiva mandala (anahata chakra), then the woman will be captivated for the whole of her life. This is said by the ascetics.

जीवेन गृह्यते जीवो जीवो जीवस्य दीयते ।
जीवस्थाने गतो जीवो बालाजीवान्तकारक: ॥ 277 ॥

277. If the woman's active swara is held by the man's active swara, and the man again puts that swara back into the active swara of the woman, he controls the woman throughout his life.

रात्र्यन्तयाम वेलायां प्रसुप्ते कामिनीजने ।
ब्रह्मजीवं पिबेद्यस्तु बालाप्राणहरो नर: ॥ 278 ॥

278. The man who drinks the sushumna swara of the woman during the period of the last yama (three hours) of the night when the woman is asleep keeps the prana of the woman captivated.

अष्टाक्षरं जपित्वा तु तस्मिन्काले गते सति ।
तत्क्षणं दीयते चन्द्रो मोहमायाति कामिनी ॥ 279 ॥

279. If, after the period of the flow of sushumna swara, one recites the eight-syllable mantra *Om Namo Narayanaya* and instantly gives his lunar swara to the woman, she develops love for him.

शयने वा प्रसङ्गे वा युवत्यालिङ्गनेऽपि वा ।
यः सूर्येण पिबेच्चन्द्रं स भवेन्मकरध्वजः ॥ 280 ॥

280. If, when sleeping or having sex or just embracing, the
man drinks the lunar swara of the woman through his
solar swara, then his charm becomes captivating like
that of Cupid.

शिव आलिङ्ग्यते शक्त्या प्रसङ्गे दक्षिणेऽपि वा ।
तत्क्षणाद्दापयेद्यस्तु   मोहयेत्कामिनीशतम् ॥ 281 ॥

281. At the time of intercourse with a woman or even during
courtship (dakshine), if the woman's active solar swara
is embraced by the man's active lunar swara, and he
immediately incites her to reciprocate his action, then
he can captivate one hundred women.

नव सप्त त्रयः पञ्च वारान्सङ्गस्तु सूर्यभे ।
चन्द्रे विद्धचतुःषट्कृत्वा वश्या भवति कामिनी ॥ 282 ॥

282. When the solar swara flows and relations take place
three, five, seven or nine times, or during the lunar
swara two, four or six times, the woman becomes
charmed and subservient.

सूर्यचन्द्रौ समाकृष्य सर्पाक्रान्त्याऽधरोष्ठयोः ।
महापद्मे मुखं स्पृष्ट्वा वारम्वारमिदं चरेत् ॥ 283 ॥

283. Drawing both his solar and lunar swaras and seizing
the lips of a woman like a serpent, one should kiss her
half-open, lotus-shaped mouth again and again.

आप्राणमिति पद्मस्य यावन्निद्रावशं गता ।
पश्चाज्जागर्ति वेलायां चोष्यते गलचक्षुषौ ॥ 284 ॥

284. The man should keep on kissing the lotus mouth of
the woman up to the full stretch of prana until she falls

asleep. Later, when it is time for her to wake up, he should kiss her on the throat and eyes.

अनेन विधिना कामी वशयेत्सर्वकामिनी: ।
इदं न वाच्यमन्यस्मिन्नित्याज्ञा परमेश्वरि ॥285॥

285. O supreme Goddess, by following these methods a man (lover) can captivate all women. But it is my order that the method of captivation should not be divulged to any other person (unworthy one).

PREGNANCY

ऋतुकालभवा नारी पञ्चमेऽह्नि यदा भवेत् ।
सूर्यचन्द्रमसोर्योगे सेवनात्पुत्र सम्भव: ॥286॥

286. If on the fifth day after the menstrual cycle when the solar swara of the man and the lunar swara of the woman is flowing, they have intercourse, then a son will be conceived.

शङ्खवल्लीं गवां दुगधे पृथ्व्यापो वहते यदा ।
भर्तुरेवं वदेद्वाक्यं पुत्रं देहि त्रिभिर्वच: ॥287॥

287. If the woman drinks shankhavalli (a herb) mixed with cow's milk, and either the earth or water element is flowing, then she should pray three times to her husband to give her a son.

ऋतुस्नाता पिबेन्नारी ऋतुदानं तु योजयेत् ।
रूपलावण्यसम्पन्नो नरसिंह: प्रसूयते ॥288॥

288. When, on completion of the menstrual cycle, the woman has taken the aforesaid drink after bathing, then the man should enter into intercourse with her. By doing so a beautiful male child as brave as a lion will be born.

सुषुम्ना सूर्यवाहेन ऋतुदानं तु योजयेत् ।
अङ्गहीनः पुमान्यस्तु जायतेऽत्रकुविग्रहः ॥ 289 ॥

289. If a man puts the flow of his solar nadi into the woman's
sushumna during relations, then a crippled and
deformed male child is produced.

विषमाङ्के दिवारात्रौ विषमाङ्के दिनाधिपः ।
चन्द्रनेत्राग्निततत्त्वेषु वन्ध्या पुत्रमवाप्नुयात् ॥ 290 ॥

290. If relations take place during the day or night after an
uneven number of days from the last day of menses,
and the man's solar swara and the woman's lunar swara
are flowing, and either the water or fire element is
active, then even a sterile woman will produce a son.

ऋत्वारम्भे रविः पुन्सां स्त्रीणां चैव सुधाकरः ।
उभयोः सङ्गमे प्राप्ते वन्ध्या पुत्रमवाप्नुयात् ॥ 291 ॥

291. If union takes place at the beginning of the fertile
period when the man's solar swara and the woman's
lunar swara are flowing, then even a sterile woman will
have a son.

ऋत्वारम्भे रविः पुन्सां शुक्रान्ते च सुधाकरः ।
अनने क्रमयोगेन नादत्ते दैवदारुकम् ॥ 292 ॥

292. If the man's solar swara flows at the start of intercourse
at the beginning of the fertile period of the woman,
and after ejaculation his lunar swara starts flowing, then
there will not be even a wooden doll in their fate (i.e.
the woman will not conceive).

चन्द्रनाडी यदा प्रश्ने गर्भे कन्या तदा भवेत् ।
सूर्यो भवेत्तदा पुत्रो द्वयोर्गर्भो विहन्यते ॥ 293 ॥

293. If one's lunar swara flows at the time of a question about pregnancy, the child will be a girl. The flow of the solar swara means it will be a boy, and if both swaras flow in sushumna. there will be a miscarriage.

पृथिव्यां पुत्री जले पुत्र: कन्यका तु प्रभञ्जने ।
तेजसि गर्भपात: स्यान्नभस्यपि नपुंसक: ॥ 294 ॥

294. If the earth element is predominant at the time of the question, then the child will be a girl; if the water element is dominant, then a boy; if air, then a girl; if fire, then an abortion; and if either, then an impotent child will be born.

चन्द्रे स्त्री पुरुष: सूर्ये मध्यमार्गे नपुंसक: ।
गर्भप्रश्ने यदा दूत: पूर्णे पुत्र: प्रजायते ॥ 295 ॥

295. The lunar swara indicates a girl, solar swara a boy, both swaras a eunuch. But if the question is asked when the messenger is on the side of the full swara, then a son will be born.

शून्ये शून्यं युगे युग्मं गर्भपातश्च सङ्क्रमे ।
तत्त्ववित्स विजानीयात्कथितं तत्तु सुन्दरी ॥ 296 ॥

296. O beautiful one, if the questioner comes to the side of the vacant (shoonya) swara, then there will be no child; if both the swaras are flowing, then twins will be born; if there is an alternation of swaras (i.e. sushumna flowing), then there will be a miscarriage. The knower of the tattwas must know what I have explained.

गर्भाधानं मारुते स्याच्च दु:खी:
दिक्षु ख्यातो वारुणे सौख्ययुक्त: ।
गर्भस्राव: स्वल्पजीवश्च वह्नौ
भोगी भव्य: पार्थिवेनार्थयुक्त: ॥ 297 ॥

297. If conception takes place when the air element is predominant, the offspring (son) will be morose; when the water element is dominant, he will be famous in all directions and will have a pleasurable life; when the fire element is dominant, there will either be an abortion or the baby will be short-lived; and when the earth element is predominant, he will enjoy material life and be handsome and wealthy.

धनवान्सौख्ययुक्तश्च   भोगवानर्थसंस्थित: ।
स्यात्रितयं वारुणे तत्त्वे व्योम्नि गर्भो विनश्यति ॥ 298 ॥

298. If conception takes place during the predominance of the water element, then the son born will be wealthy, happy and an enjoyer of material life, and his wealth will ever remain with him. If conception takes place during the dominance of the ether element, then there will be an abortion.

माहेये सुसुतोत्पत्तिर्वारुणे दुहिता भवेत् ।
शेषेषु गर्भहानि: स्याज्जातमात्रस्य वा मृति: ॥ 299 ॥

299. If conception takes place during the predominance of the earth element, then a beautiful son will be born, and under the water element a daughter. If it takes place under the other elements, then there will either be an abortion or the child will die soon after birth.

रविमध्यगतश्चन्द्रश्चन्द्रमध्यगतो   रवि: ।
ज्ञातव्यं गुरुत: शीघ्रं न वेदै: शास्त्रकोटिभि: ॥ 300 ॥

300. If the lunar swara passes through the solar swara or the solar through the lunar, then one should seek the advice of a guru quickly, because the Vedas or crores of shastras will be of no avail.

चैत्रशुक्लप्रतिपदि   प्रातस्तत्त्वविभेदत: ।
पश्यांद्विचक्षणो योगी दाक्षिणे चोत्तरायणे ॥ 301 ॥

301. The learned yogi should analyze the five elements in
the morning of the first day of Chaitra (March, April),
shukla paksha, when the sun moves to the south or
north, then ask questions about the events of the
coming year.

चन्द्रोदयस्य वेलायां वहमानोऽत्र तत्त्वत: ।
पृथिव्यापस्तथा वायु: सुभिक्षं सर्वशस्यजम् ॥ 302 ॥

302. At the time of the beginning of the moon swara, if
the earth, water or air element is active, there will be
prosperity due to abundance of grain.

तेजोव्योम्नोर्भयं घोरं दुर्भिक्षं कालतत्त्वत: ।
एवं तत्फलं ज्ञेयं वर्षे मासे दिनेष्वपि ॥ 303 ॥

303. If under the moon swara the fire or ether element
is present, then there will be serious famine and
suffering. In the same way, the effects of the tattwas
on the complete year, month or even day should be
found out.

मध्यमा भवति क्रूरा दुष्टा सर्वेषु कर्मसु ।
देशभङ्गमहारोगक्लेशकष्टादि दु:खदा ॥ 304 ॥

304. The sushumna nadi is cruel and wicked in all affairs
and causes pain through destruction of the country,
epidemics, suffering and affliction.

मेषसंक्रान्तिवेलायां स्वरभेदं विचारयेत् ।
संवत्सरफलं ब्रूयाल्लोकानां तत्त्वचिन्तक: ॥ 305 ॥

190

305. The knower of the tattwas should examine the differences in the swaras at the time of the transition of the sun into the sign of Aries and should predict results accordingly for the whole year for the benefit of the people.

पृथिव्यादिकतत्त्वेन दिनमासाब्दजं फलम् ।
शोभनं च यथा दुष्टं व्योममारुतवह्निभिः ॥ 306 ॥

306. When the earth or water element is prominent, the days, the months and the whole year will be prosperous and hold good news. If the ether, air or fire element is present, the conditions will be bad.

सुभिक्षं राष्ट्रवृद्धिः स्याद्बहुशस्या वसुन्धरा ।
बहुवृष्टिस्तथा सौख्यं पृथ्वीतत्त्वं वहेद्यदि ॥ 307 ॥

307. If at the above time (see sloka 305) the earth element is active, there will be abundant food, prosperity in the country, good crops, plentiful rain and happiness.

अतिवृष्टिः सुभिक्षं स्यादारोग्यं सौख्यमेव च ।
बहुशस्या तथा पृथ्वी अप्तत्त्वं वै वहेद्यदि ॥ 308 ॥

308. If on the above day (see sloka 305) the water element is flowing, there will be sufficient rains, abundance of food, freedom from disease, prosperity and rich crops.

दुर्भिक्षं राष्ट्रभङ्गः स्यादुत्पत्तिश्च विनश्यति ।
अल्पादल्पतरा वृष्टिरग्नितत्त्वं वहेद्यदि ॥ 309 ॥

309. If the fire element is flowing, then there will be famine, destruction of the country, destruction of the grain crops and scanty rainfall.

उत्पातोपद्रवा भीतिरल्पा वृष्टिस्युरीतयः ।
मेषसंक्रान्तिवेलायां वायुतत्त्वं वहेद्यदि ॥ 310 ॥

310. If the air element is flowing during the transition into Aries, there will be trouble, calamity, fear, scanty rainfall and natural calamity (like excess rain, rats, locusts, birds, drought, etc.).

मेषसंक्रान्तिवेलायां व्योमतत्त्वं वहेद्यदि ।
तत्रापि शून्यता ज्ञेयाशस्यादीनां सुखस्य च ॥ 311 ॥

311. During Mesha Sankranti (see sloka 305) if the ether element is active, it indicates desolation due to scanty crops and lack of prosperity.

पूर्णप्रवेशने श्वासे शस्यं तत्त्वेन सिध्यति ।
सूर्यचन्द्रेऽन्यथाभूते संग्रह: सर्वसिद्धिद: ॥ 312 ॥

312. When the full swara flows and the elements appear in their proper manner, there will be prosperity due to good crops. When the solar and lunar swaras flow unusually, then grain should be stored because there will be poor crops.

विषमे वह्नितत्त्वं स्याज्ज्ञायते केवलं नभ: ।
तत्कुर्याद्वस्तुसंग्राहो द्विमासे च महार्घता ॥ 313 ॥

313. If the fire element flows in the solar swara or only the ether element is active, there will be a steep rise in prices within two months, so one should store grain and necessary articles.

रवौ संक्रमते नाडी चन्द्रमन्ते प्रसर्पिता ।
खानिले वह्नियोगेन रौरवं जगतीतले ॥ 314 ॥

314. If the solar swara flows during the night and the lunar swara in the morning and there is a conjunction of the ether, air and fire elements, there will be a hellish condition on earth.

महीतत्त्वे स्वरोगश्च जले च जलमातृका ।
तेजसि खेटवाटीस्था शाकिनि पितृदोषत: ॥315॥

315. At the time of questioning, if the earth tattwa is active,
then know that disease is the result of prarabdha karma
(destiny). If the water element is active, disease is due
to an imbalance of the doshas. In the fire element it is
due to a disturbance of Goddess Shakini or an ancestral
fault.

आदौशून्यगतोदूत: पश्चात्पूर्णे विशेद्यदि ।
मूर्च्छितोऽपि ध्रुवं जीवेद्यद्यथं प्रतिपृच्छति ॥316॥

316. If the messenger approaches on the closed side and
sits on the side which is flowing, the sick person will
survive, even if in a coma.

यस्मिन्नङ्गे स्थितो जीवस्तत्रस्थ: परिपृच्छति ।
तदा जीवति जीवोऽसौ यदि रोगैरुपद्रुत: ॥317॥

317. If the questioner asks a question while sitting on the
side of the active swara, then the patient, though
suffering from several diseases, will survive.

दक्षिणेन यदा वायुर्दूतोरौद्राक्षरो वदेत् ।
तदा जीवति जीवोऽसौ चन्द्रे समफलं भवेत् ॥318॥

318. If the solar swara is flowing and the questioner comes
uttering terrible words, the ill person will still survive.
The results will be similar during the flow of the lunar
swara.

जीवाकारं च वा धृत्वा जीवाकारं विलोक्य च ।
जीवस्थोजीवितप्रश्ने तस्य स्याज्जीवितं फलम् ॥319॥

319. If the figure of the sick person as explained by the messenger appears on the mental screen of the swara yogi and becomes stabilized, then this indicates that the patient will survive.

वामाचारे तथा दक्षप्रवेशे यत्र वाहने ।
तत्रस्थ: पृच्छते दूतस्तस्य सिद्धिर्नसंशय: ॥ 320 ॥

320. If the messenger enters the vehicle from the right side when the lunar swara is flowing and asks a question (about a sick person) while sitting in the vehicle, his desire will undoubtedly be fulfilled.

प्रश्नेचाध: स्थितो जीवो नूनं जीवो हि जीवति ।
ऊर्ध्वचारस्थितो जीवो जीवो याति यमालयम् ॥ 321 ॥

321. If the swara flows downward at the time of questioning, the patient will be all right. If the swara flows upward, then the patient will certainly arrive at the place of Yamaraja (death).

विपरीताक्षरप्रश्ने रिक्तायां पृच्छको यदि ।
विपर्ययं च विज्ञेयं विषमस्योदये सति ॥ 322 ॥

322. If the questioner is on the side of the closed swara, his words are confused, and the uneven swara begins to flow, the results will be reversed.

चन्द्रस्थाने स्थितो जीवो सूर्यस्थाने तु पृच्छक: ।
तदा प्राणाद्रियुक्तोऽसौ यद्यपि वैद्यशतैर्वृत: ॥ 323 ॥

323. If the lunar swara is flowing and the questioner sits on the side of the solar swara (i.e. the right side), then the patient will die even if attended to by hundreds of physicians.

पिङ्गलायां स्थितो जीवो वामे दूतस्तु पृच्छति ।
तदाऽपि प्रियते रोगी यदि त्राता महेश्वरः ॥ 324 ॥

324. If pingala is active and the messenger asks a question
from the left, then even after having Shiva's protection
the sick person will not survive.

एकस्य भूतस्य विपर्ययेण रोगाभिभूतिर्भवतीह पुंसाम् ।
तयोर्द्वयोर्बन्धुसुहृद्विपत्तिः पक्षद्वये व्यत्ययतो मृतिः स्यात् ॥ 325 ॥

325. When one element flows out of order, it indicates
suffering caused by disease. When two elements flow
out of order, it indicates a bad omen for relatives and
friends. When the elements flow out of order for one
month continually, death is certain.

TIME

मासादौ चैव पक्षादौ वत्सरादौ यथाक्रमम् ।
क्षयकालं परीक्षेत वायुचारवशात् सुधीः ॥ 326 ॥

326. On the basis of the flow of swara a wise person should
examine the time of death in the beginning of the
month, fortnight and year in the same order.

पञ्चभूतात्मकं दीपं शिवस्नेहेन सिञ्चितम् ।
रक्षयेत्सूर्यवातेन प्राणजीवः स्थिरोभवेत् ॥ 327 ॥

327. This body consisting of the five elements is like an
earthen lamp (deepaka) nourished by the oil of Shiva
(prana) and the life of that person who protects it from
the wind of the sun (solar swara) becomes stabilized.

मारुतं बन्धयित्वा तु सूर्यं बन्धयते यदि ।
अभ्यासाज्जीवते जीवः सूर्यकालेऽपि वञ्चिते ॥ 328 ॥

195

328. A person who regularly avoids the solar swara throughout the day (i.e. from sunrise to sunset) by controlling
the breath flow (through pranayama, etc.) enjoys long
life.

गगनात्स्त्रवते चन्द्र: कायपद्मानि सिञ्चयेत् ।
कर्मयोगसदाभ्यासैरमर: शशिसंश्रयात् ॥ ३२९ ॥

329. The moon flows down from the sky (i.e. bindu). One
should nourish the body lotuses (chakras) with the
nectar flowing from bindu. With the thorough practice
of karma yoga and nourishment from the nectar flow,
one becomes immortal.

शशाङ्कं वारयेद्रात्रौ दिवावार्यो दिवाकर: ।
इत्यभ्यासरतो नित्यं सयोगी नात्रसंशय: ॥ ३३० ॥

330. One who always avoids the flow of ida at night, and
pingala during the day, becomes a perfected yogi.
About this, there is no doubt.

DEATH PREDICTIONS

अहोरात्रं यदैकत्र वहते यस्य मारुत: ।
तदा तस्य भवेन्मृत्यु: सम्पूर्णे वत्सरत्रये ॥ ३३१ ॥

331. When the flow of the swara is continuous night and
day through one nostril, his death will come in three
years.

अहोरात्रद्वयं यस्य पिङ्गलायां सदा गति: ।
तस्य वर्षद्वयं प्रोक्तं जीवितं तत्त्ववेदिभि: ॥ ३३२ ॥

332. If the solar swara of a person flows continuously for two
consecutive days and nights, it is said by the knowers
of the elements that he has only two years of life
remaining.

त्रिरात्रं वहते यस्य वायुरेकपुटे स्थितः ।
तदा संवत्सरायुस्तं प्रवदन्ति मनीषिणः ॥ ३३३ ॥

333. When the same nadi flows continuously for up to three
nights, one year is left for him to live, the wise say.

रात्रौ चन्द्रो दिवा सूर्यो वहेद्यस्य निरन्तरम् ।
जानीयात्तस्य वै मृत्युः षण्मासाभ्यन्तरे भवेत् ॥ ३३४ ॥

334. When the lunar swara of a person flows continuously at
night and the solar swara during the day, his death will
definitely come in six months.

INDICATIONS OF DEATH

लक्ष्यं लक्षितलक्षणेन सलिले भानुर्यदा दृश्यते
क्षीणो दक्षिणपश्चिमोत्तरपुरः षट्त्रिद्विमासैकतः ।
मध्ये छिद्रमिदं भवेद्दशदिनं धूमाकुलं तद्दिने
सर्वज्ञैरपि भाषितं मुनिवरैरायुः प्रमाणं स्फुटम् ॥३३५॥

335. If, when looking at the reflection of the sun in water,
one finds the sun's disc cut or missing in the southern,
western, northern or eastern direction, one will die
within six, three, two or one month respectively. If one
finds a hole in the centre of the reflection, one will
die in ten days. If the sun is seen to be covered with
smoke, one will die on the same day. The omniscient
great sages have clearly spoken thus about the span of
one's life.

EXAMINING THE MESSENGER

दूतः रक्तकषायकृष्णवसनो दन्तक्षतो मुण्डित-
स्तैलाभ्यक्तशरीर रज्जुककरो दीनोऽश्रुपूर्णोत्तरः ।
भस्माङ्गारकपालपाशमुसली सूर्यास्तमायाति यः
कालीशून्यपदस्थितो गदयुतः कालानलस्यादृतः ॥ ३३६ ॥

336. If the one coming to ask about a sick person is wearing red, saffron or black-coloured clothes, has broken teeth, a shaved head, oil smeared on his body, a rope in his hand, looks miserable, is in tears, comes to the left side, has ashes, burning embers, a skull, noose or a pestle in his hand, or comes after sunset, he has come in the form of Yamaraja for the sick person (i.e. the sick person will die).

अकस्माच्चित्तविकृतिरकस्मात्पुरुषोत्तमः ।
अकस्मादिन्द्रियोत्पातः सन्निपाताग्रलक्षणम् ॥337॥

337. If the sick person suddenly gets worse and suddenly feels all right or the senses suddenly become confused, understand these are the symptoms of delirium.

शरीरं शीतलं यस्य प्रकृतिर्विकृता भवेत् ।
तदरिष्टं समासेन व्यासतस्तु निबोधये ॥338॥

338. I will describe separately (point wise) and in brief the unfavourable symptoms of a sick person approaching death whose body has become cold and the temperament has become unnatural.

दुष्टशब्देषुरमतेऽशुद्धशब्देषु चाप्यति ।
पश्चातापो भवेद्यस्य तस्यमृत्युर्नसंशयः ॥339॥

339. One who is pleased with foul language and feels happiness in speaking incorrect words and later repents over it will die soon, there is no doubt about it.

हुङ्कारः शीतलो यस्य फूत्कारो वह्निसन्निभः ।
महावैद्यो भवेद्यस्य तस्यमृत्युर्भवेद्ध्रुवम् ॥340॥

340. One whose humkara (i.e. forceful exhalation through the nose with a loud sound of hum) is cold and whose

phootkara (i.e. forceful blowing through the mouth) is hot like fire is sure to die even though being attended by eminent physicians.

जिह्वां विष्णुपदं ध्रुवं सुरपदं सन्मातृकामण्डलम्
एतान्येवमरुन्धतीममृतगुं शुक्रं ध्रुवं वा क्षणम् ।
एतेष्वेकमपि स्फुटं न पुरुष: पश्येत्पुर: प्रेषित:
सोऽवश्यं विशतीह कालवदनं सम्वत्सरादूर्ध्वत: ॥ ३४१ ॥

341. The person who cannot see even one of the following clearly present before him: his own tongue, the sky, the Pole Star, the Milky Way, the Matrika Mandala (a particular constellation of stars), Arundhati (a tiny star close to one of the stars of the big bear), the moon, the morning star or the centre of a circle, will definitely die within a year.

SIGNS OF DEATH

अरश्मिबिम्बं सूर्यस्य वह्ने: शीतांशुमालिन: ।
दृष्ट्वैकादशमासायुर्नरश्चोर्ध्वं न जीवति ॥ ३४२ ॥

342. One who cannot see the disc of the rising or setting sun (without rays), or the disc of the moon, or fire will not live beyond eleven months.

वाप्यां पुरीषमूत्राणि सुवर्णं रजतं तथा ।
प्रत्यक्षमथवा स्वप्ने दशमासान्न जीवति ॥ ३४३ ॥

343. One who either in the waking state or in a dream sees human excreta, urine, gold or silver in a pond will not live beyond ten months.

क्वचित्पश्यति यो दीपं सुवर्णं च कषान्वितम् ।
विरूपाणि च भूतानि नवमासान्न जीवति ॥ ३४४ ॥

344. One who does not see the glow of a lamp or gold rubbed on a touchstone, or who sees all living beings in deformed shapes, does not live longer than nine months.

स्थूलाङ्गोऽपि कृश: कृशोऽपिसहसा स्थूलत्वमालभ्यते
प्राप्तो वा कनकप्रभां यदि भवेत्क्रूरोऽपि कृष्णच्छवि: ।
शूरो भीरुसुधीरधर्मनिपुण: शान्तो विकारी पुमा-
नित्येवं प्रकृति: प्रयाति चलनं मासाष्टकं जीवति ॥345॥

345. If a fat person suddenly becomes thin or a thin person becomes fat, or if his glittering golden complexion suddenly becomes rough and black, or his nature suddenly changes from bravery to cowardice, from piety to impiety, from steadiness to fickleness, then he will live only up to eight months.

पीडाभवेत्पाणितले च जिह्वा-
मूले तथास्याद्रुधिरं च कृष्णम् ।
विद्धं न च ग्लायति यत्र दष्ट्या
जीवेन्मनुष्य: स हि सप्तमासम् ॥346॥

346. If one feels pain in the palm or at the root of the tongue, or if the blood becomes blackish, or if one does not even look towards the place where pricked, then one will live up to seven months.

मध्याङ्गुलीनां त्रितयं न वक्रं
रोगं विना शुष्यति यस्य कण्ठ: ।
मुहुर्मुहु: प्रश्नवशेन जाड्यात्
षड्भि: स मासै: प्रलयं प्रयाति ॥347॥

347. If the middle three fingers do not bend, if without sickness the throat becomes dry, and if there appears to be loss of memory by asking questions again and again, then his death will come in six months.

न यस्य स्मरणं किञ्चिद्विद्यते भूतकर्मणि ।
सोऽवश्यं पञ्चमे मासे स्कन्धारूढो भविष्यति ॥ ३४८ ॥

348. One who does not remember anything of the past will surely die in five months.

यस्य न स्फुरति ज्योतिः पीड्यते नयनद्वयम् ।
मरणं तस्य निर्दिष्टं चतुर्थेमासे निश्चितम् ॥ ३४९ ॥

349. One whose eyes have no palpitation but have pain in both is bound to die in four months.

दन्ताश्च वृषणौ यस्य न किञ्चिदपि पीड्यते ।
तृतीयमासतोऽवश्यं कालाज्ञायां भवेत्नरः ॥ ३५० ॥

350. One whose teeth and scrotum do not experience any pain (when pressed) will surely die in three months.

CHHAYOPASANA

कालो दूरस्थितो वापि येनोपायेन लक्ष्यते ।
तं वदामि समासेन यथाऽऽदिष्टंशिवागमे ॥ ३५१ ॥

351. Now I will describe in brief the science as directed in the Shivashastra by which distant death also could be indicated.

एकान्तं विजनं गत्वा कृत्वाऽऽदित्यं च पृष्ठतः ।
निरीक्षयेत्निजच्छायां कण्ठदेशे समाहितः ॥ ३५२ ॥

352. Going alone to a lonely place and keeping the sun on his back, one should concentrate his attention on the throat area of his shadow.

ततश्चाकाशमीक्षेत ह्रीं परब्रह्मणे नमः ।
अष्टोत्तरशतं जप्त्वा ततः पश्यति शङ्करम् ॥ ३५३ ॥

353. Then he should look towards the sky uttering the mantra *Hrim Parabrahmane Namah* one hundred and eight times, then the form of Shiva is seen.

शुद्धस्फटिक सङ्कशं नानारूपधरं हरम् ।
षण्मासाभ्यासयोगेन भूचराणां पतिर्भवेत् ।
वर्षद्वयेन तेनाथ कर्ताहर्ता स्वयं प्रभुः ॥ ३५४ ॥

354. He will see Lord Shiva whose appearance is like pure crystal and who assumes numerous forms. He who practises this upasana for six months becomes a king, and if he continues to practise for two years, he may himself become the creator, destroyer and all-powerful Lord.

त्रिकालज्ञत्वमाप्नोति परमानन्दमेव च ।
सतताभ्यासयोगेन नास्ति किञ्चित्सुदुर्लभम् ॥ ३५५ ॥

355. Through regular constant practice he will become the knower of all the three times, kalas, (i.e. past, present and future) and will get absolute bliss. Nothing will remain inaccessible to him.

तद्रूपं कृष्णवर्णं यः पश्यति व्योम्नि निर्मले ।
षण्मासान्मृत्युमाप्नोति स योगी नात्रसंशयः ॥ ३५६ ॥

356. The practitioner (or yogi) who sees within the clear sky the form of Shiva as black-coloured will undoubtedly die in six months.

पीतेव्याधिर्भयं रक्ते नीले हानिं विनिर्दिशेत् ।
नानावर्णोऽथ चेत्तस्मिन् सिद्धिश्च गीयते महान् ॥ ३५७ ॥

357 If the complexion of the form of Shiva appears to him as yellow, he will suffer from disease; if red, he will suffer from fear; if blue, he will undergo loss; and

if multicoloured, he will achieve success or siddhis (supernatural powers).

पदे गुल्फे च जठरे तु विनाश: क्रमशो भवेत् ।
विनश्यतो यदा बाहू स्वयं तु म्रियते ध्रुवम् ॥358॥

358. If he sees that the feet, ankles and belly are missing from the form of Shiva, then he will meet gradual destruction, and when he sees both arms missing, he himself will definitely die.

वामबाहुस्तदा भार्या नश्येदिति न संशय: ।
दक्षिणे बन्धुनाशो हि मृत्युर्मासे विनिर्दिशेत् ॥359॥

359. If he sees that the left arm of the form of Shiva is missing, then his wife will undoubtedly die, and if he sees that the right arm is missing, then his kinsmen will die, and in a month's time he himself will die.

अशिरो मासमरणं विनाजङ्घे दिनाष्टकम् ।
अष्टभि: स्कन्धनाशेनच्छायालोपेन तत्क्षणात् ॥360॥

360. If he does not see the head of the form, he will die within a month. If he does not see the thighs or shoulders, he will die within eight days. If he does not see the shadow of the form at all, then he will die that very moment.

प्रात: पृष्ठगते रवौ च निमिषाच्छायाऽङ्गुलिश्चाधरं
दृष्ट्वाऽर्द्धेन मृतिस्त्वनन्तरमहोच्छायां नर: पश्यति ।
तत्कर्णाँसकरास्य पार्श्वहृदयाभावे क्षणार्धात्स्वयं
दिङ्मूढो हि नर: शिरोविगमतो मासांस्तु षड्जीवति ॥361॥

361. In the morning, stand with the sun at one's back and concentrate on the shadow. If the fingers and the lips are missing, then death will be immediate. One who is unable to see 'is own shadow can expect death within

a moment. If one does not see the ears, shoulders, hands, face, sides or chest, then death can come in half a second. If the shadow is headless and one does not know the significance of the different directions, then one will live only up to six months.

एकादिषोडशाहानि यदि भानुर्निरन्तरम् ।
वहेद्यस्य च वै मृत्यु: शेषाहेन च मासिके ॥ 362 ॥

362. If the solar swara flows for sixteen days continuously, death will come by the end of the even days of the month.

सम्पूर्णं वहते सूर्यश्चन्द्रमा नैव दृश्यते ।
पक्षेण जायते मृत्यु: कालज्ञेनानुभाषितम् ॥ 363 ॥

363. If the solar swara flows full strength constantly and the lunar swara does not flow at all, death will occur within fifteen days. This is said by the wise who have knowledge of time.

मूत्रं पुरीषं वायुश्च समकालं प्रवर्त्तते ।
तदाऽसौ चलितो ज्ञेयो दशाहे म्रियते ध्रुवम् ॥ 364 ॥

364. When urine, excreta and wind are all expelled simultaneously, then he is a lost case and he will surely die within ten days.

सम्पूर्ण वहते चन्द्र: सूर्यो नैव च दृश्यते ।
मासेन जायते मृत्यु: कालज्ञेनानुभाषितम् ॥ 365 ॥

365. If the lunar swara flows full strength constantly and the solar swara does not flow at all, death will occur within a month. This is said by the wise who have knowledge of time.

अरुन्धतीं ध्रुवं चैव विष्णोस्त्रीणि पदानि च ।
आयुर्हीना न पश्यन्ति चतुर्थं मातृमण्डलम् ॥ 366 ॥

366. Those whose duration of life has come to an end are
unable to see the stars Arundhati, Dhruva, Matrika
Mandala and the sky.

अरुन्धती भवेज्जिह्वा ध्रुवोनासाग्रमेव च ।
भ्रुवौ विष्णुपदं ज्ञेयं तारकं मातृमण्डलम् ॥ 367 ॥

367. In the above sloka the tongue represents Arundhati,
the tip of the nose Dhruva, the eyebrows the feet of
Vishnu and the stars the Matrika Mandala (i.e. the
seven divine mothers).

नव भ्रुवं सप्त घोषं पञ्च तारां त्रिनासिकाम् ।
जिह्वामेकदिनं प्रोक्तं म्रियते मानवो ध्रुवम् ॥ 368 ॥

368. The man will surely die in nine days who is unable to
see his eyebrows, in seven days if he is unable to hear
any sound, in five days if he is unable to see the stars,
in three days if he is unable to see his nose and in one
day if he is unable to see his tongue.

कोणावक्ष्णोरङ्गुलिभ्यां किञ्चत्पीड्य निरीक्षयेत् ।
यदा न दृश्यते बिन्दुर्दशाहेन भवेन्मृतः ॥ 369 ॥

369. If after pressing the corners of the eyes slightly with
the fingers and gazing steadfastly at a blank space,
one does not see any spot of light, one will die within
ten days.

तीर्थस्नानेन दानेन तपसा सुकृतेन च ।
जपैर्ध्यानेन योगेन जायते कालवञ्चना ॥ 370 ॥

370. Death can be averted by bathing in the holy places
(tirthas), by performing charity, penance, austerity

or virtuous acts, recitation of mantras or prayers, meditation and yoga.

शरीरं नाशयन्त्येते दोषा धातुमलास्तथा ।
समस्तु वायुर्विज्ञेयो बलतेजोविवर्धनः ॥ 371 ॥

371. The disorders of the three humors (i.e. vata, pitta and kapha), the primary fluids and the excretions (twelve in number) of the body keep on destroying it. But the balancing of the vayu (wind) increases vigour and strength.

रक्षणीयस्ततो देहो यतो धर्मादिसाधनम् ।
योगाभ्यासात्समायान्ति साधुयाप्यास्तु साध्यताम् ।
असाध्याः जीवितं घ्नन्ति न तत्रास्ति प्रतिक्रिया ॥ 372 ॥

372. Therefore, the body must be protected (i.e. kept healthy) because the body is the primary means for performing religious duties. By practising yoga the virtuous as well as the contemptible come to the curable state of their diseases or ailments. The ailments which become incurable due to not practising yoga kill afflicted persons because there is no other remedy.

येषां हृदि स्फुरति शाश्वतमद्वितीयं
तेजस्तमोनिवहनाशकरं रहस्यम् ।
तेषामखण्डशशिरम्यसुकान्तिभाजां
स्वप्नेऽपि नो भवति कालभयं नराणाम् ॥ 373 ॥

373. There is no fear of death even in dream to such persons whose hearts throb with the mystic incantation of the eternal and unparalleled knowledge of the swara, which destroys a multitude of dark ignorance and illumines them like the full moon.

SECTION ON SAMADHI

इडा गङ्गेति विज्ञेया पिङ्गला यमुना नदी ।
मध्ये सरस्वती विद्यात्प्रयागादिसमस्तथा ॥374॥

374. Ida nadi is known as Ganga, pingala as Yamuna, and the central nadi (sushumna) as Saraswati, and the place of their confluence is known as Prayag.

आदौ साधनमाख्यातं सद्यः प्रत्ययकारकम् ।
बद्धपद्मासनो योगी बन्धयेदुड्डियानकम् ॥375॥

375. In the beginning the means of accomplishing the practices is told to generate instant confidence. Now the practitioner sitting in the lotus posture should practise uddiyana bandha (i.e. retain the apana air at the navel).

पूरकः कुम्भकश्चैव रेचकश्च तृतीयकः ।
ज्ञातव्यो योगिभिर्नित्यं देहसंशुद्धिहेतवे ॥376॥

376. In order to purify their bodies yogis should know thoroughly about (the aspects of pranayama which are) puraka (inhalation), kumbhaka (retention) and rechaka (exhalation).

पूरकः कुरुते वृद्धि धातुसाम्यं तथैव च ।
कुम्भके स्तम्भनं कुर्याज्जीवरक्षाविवर्द्धनम् ॥377॥

377. Puraka is responsible for the growth and harmony of the essential ingredients of the body, whereas kumbhaka enhances the preservation of life that is performed by suspension of the breath.

रेचको हरते पापं कुर्याद्योगपदं व्रजेत् ।
पश्चात्सङ्ग्रामवतिष्ठेल्लयबन्धं च कारयेत् ॥378॥

378. Rechaka destroys all evils of the mind and physical impurities and the practitioner attains the status of yogi. Thus, after completion of rechaka the practitioner should remain steady and repeat the above practice rhythmically with deep concentration.

कुम्भयेत्सहजं वायुं यथाशक्ति प्रकल्पयेत् ।
रेचयेच्चन्द्रमार्गेण   सूर्येणापूरयेत्सुधी: ॥379॥

379. The wise should inhale through the right nostril and perform kumbhaka, retaining the breath and prana to the extent of their capacity, and then exhale through the left nostril.

चन्द्रं पिबति सूर्यश्च सूर्यं पिबति चन्द्रमा: ।
अन्योन्यकालभावेन जीवेदाचन्द्रतारकम् ॥380॥

380. One who breathes through the right (sun) channel when it is time for the left (moon) and then breathes through the left channel when it is time for the right (i.e. by breathing through the channel which is not active) will live as long as the moon and the stars exist.

स्वीयाङ्गे वहते नाडी तन्नाडीरोधनं कुरु ।
मुखबन्धममुञ्चन्वै पवनं जायते युवा ॥381॥

381. One who restrains the active nadi which is flowing through its own channel by closing its mouth (entrance) and by not releasing the flow of air, certainly achieves youthfulness.

मुखनासाक्षिकर्णान्तानङ्गुलीभिर्निरोधयेत् ।
तत्त्वोदयमिति ज्ञेयं षण्मुखीकरणं प्रियम् ॥382॥

382. Close the mouth, nostrils, eyes and ears with four fingers and become aware of the active tattwa. This is the pleasant shanmukhi mudra.

तस्य रूपं गति: स्वादो मण्डलं लक्षणं त्विदम् ।
स वेत्ति मानवो लोके संसर्गादपि मार्गवित् ॥383॥

383. Such a man who becomes acquainted with the paths
of the elements by practising shanmukhi mudra also
acquires knowledge of the form, motion, taste, region
and attribute. Knowledge about the tattwas is also
obtained by establishing an intimate relation with them
through regular practice.

निराशो निष्कलो योगी न किञ्चिदपि चिन्तयेत् ।
वासनामुन्मनां कृत्वा कालं जयति लीलया ॥384॥

384. The desireless and sinless yogi should not worry about
anything. By making himself free from the impressions
unconsciously left on his mind by past good or bad
actions, which therefore produce pleasure or pain, he
can effortlessly obtain victory over death.

विश्वस्य वेदिकाशक्तिर्नेत्राभ्यां परिदृश्यते ।
तत्रस्थं तु मनो यस्य याममात्रं भवेदिह ॥385॥

385. The power of knowing the whole world is experienced
through the eyes by the person whose mind becomes
stable in that power even for one yama (three hours).

तस्यायुर्वर्धते नित्यं घटिकात्रयमानत: ।
शिवेनोक्तं पुरा तन्त्रे सिद्धस्य गुणगह्वरे ॥386॥

386. Then the life of such a person goes on increasing at the
rate of three ghatikas every day, Shiva has said in olden
times in the tantra shastras, which is in the hidden
knowledge of siddhas.

बद्ध्वा पद्मासनं ये गुदगतपवनं सन्निरुद्ध्याप्तमुच्चै:
तं तस्यापानरन्ध्रेक्रमजितमनिलं प्राणशक्त्या निरुद्ध्य ।

एकीभूतं सुषुम्नाविवरमुपगतं ब्रह्मरन्ध्रे च नीत्वा
निक्षिप्याकाशमार्गे शिवचरणरता यान्ति ते केऽपि धन्याः ॥ 387 ॥

387. Yogis, sitting in padmasana, should stop the apana vayu situated in the anal region, raise it upwards and then merge it with the prana vayu. When both vayus have merged and reached sushumna nadi opening, they should be taken through the Brahmarandhra and released in the path of the sky. This is achieved only by a few blessed ones who are devoted to the feet of Shiva.

एतज्जानाति यो योगी एतत्पठति नित्यशः ।
सर्वदुःखविनिर्मुक्तो लभते वाञ्छितं फलम् ॥ 388 ॥

388. The yogi who knows this text and chants it every day puts an end to all his sorrows and his desires are fulfilled.

स्वरज्ञानं नरे यत्र लक्ष्मीः पदतले भवेत् ।
सर्वत्र च शरीरेऽपि सुखं तस्य सदा भवेत् ॥ 389 ॥

389. The one who is master of the science of swara has Lakshmi (prosperity, good fortune) living at his feet, and he is ever and everywhere happy and also physically comfortable.

प्रणवः सर्ववेदानां ब्राह्मणे भास्करो यथा ।
मृत्युलोके तथा पूज्यः स्वरज्ञानी पुमानपि ॥ 390 ॥

390. Just as Omkara is revered by all the Vedas and surya (the sun) by the Brahmanas, the man who has knowledge of the swara is worshipped by the people of this transitory world.

नाडीत्रयं विजानाति तत्त्वज्ञानं तथैव च ।
नैव तेन भवेत्तुल्यं लक्षकोटिरसायनम् ॥ 391 ॥

391. Even lakhs or crores of the elixir of life cannot equal a person who has complete knowledge of the three nadis and of the tattwas.

एकाक्षरप्रदातारं   नाडीभेदविवेचकम् ।
पृथिव्यां नास्ति तद्द्रव्यं यद्दत्वा चानृणी भवेत् ॥ 392 ॥

392. There is nothing on the earth with which one can repay and be free from the debt of the person having discriminatory knowledge of the nadis, swaras and tattwas and a teacher of even one letter of that knowledge.

स्वरतत्त्वं तथा युद्धं देवि वश्यं स्त्रियस्तथा ।
गर्भाधानं च रोगश्च कलार्द्धेनैवमुच्यते ॥ 393 ॥

393. O Goddess! Through the knowledge of the Swarodaya shastra, the details and predictions about the swaras, tattwas, wars, captivation of women, conception and disease can be had in half a kala (a small measure of time) only.

एवं प्रवर्तितं लोके प्रसिद्धं सिद्धयोगिभि: ।
चन्द्रार्कग्रहणे जाप्यं पठतां सिद्धिदायकम् ॥ 394 ॥

394. Thus the science of Swarodaya was founded in this world and it was propagated by yogis who had achieved perfection. Its recitation during the lunar and solar eclipses and also its mere reading provides siddhis.

एवं प्रवर्तितं लोके प्रसिद्धं सिद्धयोगिभि: ।
चन्द्रार्कग्रहणे जाप्यं पठतां सिद्धिदायकम् ॥ 395 ॥

395. Being at one's own place of living and practising abstinence in food and sleep, one (the practitioner of swara yoga) should keep thinking about and concentrating on Paramatma, the Supreme Power. One will

then be blessed with the power that whatever one perceives will happen (come true).

इति श्री शिवपार्वतीसंवादे स्वरोदयशास्त्रं समाप्तम् ।

Thus ends the Swarodaya shastra in the form of a dialogue between Shiva and Parvati.

Appendices

Glossary

Adinath – name given to Lord Shiva by the natha sect of yogis; first guru of the natha yogis; the primordial guru of all; cosmic consciousness

Agni tattwa – fire element

Ahamkara – ego; awareness of the existence of 'I'; centre of individual, mental, emotional, psychic and physical functioning

Ajapa japa – spontaneous repetition of mantra

Ajna chakra – psychic and pranic centre situated at the medulla oblongata; seat of intuition; third eye; eye of Shiva; centre of command or monitoring centre

Akasha tattwa – ether element

Alambusha nadi – situated in kandasthan, the coccygeal plexus

Amavasya – fifteenth day of the dark fortnight when there is absolutely no moon visible

Amrita – psychic nectar causing one to feel intoxication and bliss; mrit means death, amrit, means beyond death

Anahata chakra – psychic and pranic centre situated in the region of the heart and cardiac plexus; fourth chakra in human evolution

Angula – specific measurement, the width of one finger

Apa or apas – water element

Apana vayu – pranic air current operating in the lower abdominal region, causing elimination through the excretory and reproductive organs

Asana – traditionally a comfortable meditative sitting pose, also a specific position of the body for channelling prana

215

Ashtami – eighth day of the moon's phase occurring once a fortnight

Ashubha – inauspicious

Atma soul or inner spirit; the universal atma (paramatma) manifests as the individual atma (jivatma)

Atma anubhuti – anubhuti means experience or experienced; therefore, it is the experience of the atma

Aum – cosmic vibration of the universe

Bhu loka – terrestrial plane of existence

Bhumi tattwa – earth element, see prithvi tattwa

Bhuva loka – intermediate realm between earth and heaven

Bija mantra – seed mantra

Brahma – universal creator; one of the three aspects of the universal self; in the physical body it is the creative power of mooladhara chakra

Brahma nadi – finest nadi inside sushumna representing the state of turiya

Brihadaranyaka Upanishad – generally recognized as the most important Upanishad, discussing the identity of the individual atma in relation to the universal self, different modes of worship, religion and meditation

Buddhi – intellect, mental faculty of intelligence

Chakra – circle, wheel, psychic centre in the pranic body; conjunction point of nadis

Chandra – moon

Chandra nadi – ida nadi

Chandra swara – flow of breath through the left nostril, indicating activation of ida nadi

Chaturthi – fourth day of the moon's phase occurring once a fortnight

Chidakasha – psychic space in front of the closed eyes, just behind the forehead

Chit – consciousness

Chitra or chitrini nadi – third nadi inside sushumna

Chitta – individual consciousness, including the conscious, subconscious and unconscious layers of mind

Dakshina swara – right nostril activities when the flow of air is coming from the right nostril only, signifying an active pingala nadi

216

Dashami – tenth day of the moon's phase; occurs twice a month

Devadatta – pranic air current causing yawning

Dhananjaya – one of the upa pranas which remains in the body after death

Dharana – technique of concentration; stage when the mind is fully one-pointed or concentrated

Dhatu – minerals of the body

Dhyana – meditation; state of introversion of mind where the meditator and object of meditation come in close range of each other

Dwitiya – second day of the moon's phase occurring once a fortnight

Ekadashi – eleventh day of the moon's phase, considered to be very important because it has a strong effect on the body and mind; in India fasting is recommended on this date or tithi

Gandhari nadi – behind ida, running from the left eye to the left leg

Ganga – also known as Ganges; famous holy river in India having spiritual, religious and esoteric significance; also symbolizes ida nadi

Ghati – period of 24 minutes, 1/60 of 24 hours

Gorakhnath – famous tantric guru, disciple of Matsyendranath, founder of the natha school of hatha yoga, and second in the line of the eighty-four siddhas

Guna – quality of nature; threefold capacity of nature or prakriti (see tamas, rajas and sattwa)

Guru – spiritually enlightened soul who by the light of his own atma can dispel darkness, ignorance and illusion of the mind, and enlighten the soul of his disciple or devotee

Guru chakra – ajna chakra, corresponding to the pineal gland in the physical body

Ham-So – Shiva or pure consciousness; hamsa means swan which has the unique ability to extract pure milk from a mixture of milk and water; when the mantra Ham-So is perfected, one can perceive the pure reality or essence of creation; Ham-So is also the psychic sound and mantra of the breath, (see So-Ham)

Hastijihva nadi – pranic channel running in front and to one side of ida nadi

Hiranyagarbha – literally golden womb or egg; where the creation of the universe begins when Shiva and Shakti, consciousness and energy, live together but creation is not yet manifest

Hridayakasha – psychic space of the heart centre

Ida nadi – major nadi running on the left side of the body through which manasa shakti passes; some opinions hold that ida emerges from mooladhara and runs straight to ajna chakra, but it is mostly believed that ida emanates from mooladhara and then intersects and crosses all the intermediate chakras before reaching ajna; represents the internal worlds and subconscious mind

Jagrat – conscious, waking state of reality

Jagrit – conscious, awake

Jagriti – conscious realm, material world of the senses

Jala tattwa – water element, apas

Jihva nadi – upward flowing nadi (position not stated in the Upanishads)

Jiva – individual life

Jivatma – individual soul

Jnana – same as gyana; cognition or knowledge, wisdom

Jnanendriya – the five senses of knowledge: ears, eyes, nose, tongue and skin

Kandasthana – conjunction point of the nadis in either mooladhara or manipura

Karana sharira – causal body

Karma – action, deed; law of action and reaction

Karmashaya – the storage of past impressions, deeds, words and thoughts

Karmendriya – five organs of action: hands, feet, speech, excretory and reproductive organs

Kosha – sheath of the body and mind, realm of experience

Krikara vayu – pranic air current stimulating hunger, thirst, sneezing and coughing

Krishna paksha – black fortnight when the moon is waning

Kuhu nadi – lying in front of sushumna

Kumbhaka – breath retention

Kundalini – man's spiritual energy, capacity and consciousness, also known as the serpent power, because when it is awakened and the energy travels through sushumna, up the vertebral column, an inner sound can be heard like the hissing of a snake

Kurma nadi – situated below the throat pit, in the shape of an inverted tortoise; according to Patanjali, when you practise and perfect samyama on this nadi, you become firm and immovable, mentally, physically, emotionally and psychically

Kurma vayu – pranic air current causing the eyelids to blink

Lakshmi – goddess of wealth, consort of Vishnu, and the power of manipura chakra; in the swara texts it says that swara yoga is safeguarded by Lakshmi, which implies that through the practice of swara yoga the faculties of manipura chakra are awakened, the pranas are stimulated to preserve and take care of all the body's necessities and one will never want materially

Maha nadi – sushumna

Mahat – cosmic consciousness

Mala – garland or rosary of a particular type of bead, either 108, 54, 27 beads or the number specified by the guru; beads can be made of tulsi wood, sandal, rudraksha, coral, crystal or other precious stones, usually for practising japa or mantra sadhana; flower malas are also offered to the guru

Manas – mind, finite mind, mundane mental activity

Manasa shakti – mental energy channelled through ida nadi

Manomaya kosha – sheath made of mind and thought

Mantra – particular subtle sound vibration; process of liberating energy and consciousness from the shackles of the mind

Maran – a rite performed for the purpose of destroying an enemy

Mohan – a magical charm employed to bewilder an enemy

Mooladhara chakra – lowest psychic and pranic centre in human evolution, situated in the perineum

Mudra – physical/mental/psychic attitude of mind and body which channels the cosmic energy

219

Nada – subtle sound vibration

Nadi – river; pranic flow of shakti

Naga vayu – pranic air current which induces belching

Naumi – ninth day of the moon's phase, occurring once a fortnight

Om – the cosmic vibration of the universe, universal mantra; same as Aum; represents four states of mind: conscious, subconscious, unconscious and universal or cosmic mind

Paksha – fortnight

Panchami – fifth day of moon's phase, occurring once a fortnight

Pancha tattwa – the five elements: earth, water, fire, air and ether

Paramatma – the greatest atma, universal self

Pawan tattwa – air element, vayu tattwa

Payaswini nadi – terminating at right big toe, between poosha and behind pingala nadis

Pingala nadi – main nadi on the right side of the body conducting prana shakti, emerging opposite ida on the right side of mooladhara chakra and intersecting each of the chakras until it reaches ajna chakra; also associated with the mundane realm of existence and conscious experiences

Pooraka – inhalation

Poornima – full moon day

Poosha nadi – behind pingala, running from the right eye to the abdomen

Prajna – intuition

Prana – vital energy force sustaining life and creation, which permeates the whole of creation; existing in both the macro and microcosmos

Prana vayu – pranic air currents; general name of all the vayus; also particular function of vayu in the thoracic region

Pranayama – breathing technique which increases the pranic capacity store

Prathama – first day of the moon's phases

Prithvi tattwa – earth element

Rajas – second quality of nature; dynamism, movement, oscillating state of mind

Rudra – name given to Lord Shiva in the Vedas, also indicates the first aspect of nature, tamas; generally Rudra signifies transformation through destruction; Rudra is said to have sprung from Brahma's forehead and is one of the holy trinity

Sadashiva – purified and subtle state of consciousness; sadashiva is said to reside in vishuddhi chakra; when the consciousness is awakened in this centre by kundalini shakti, the mind is purified

Sadhaka – spiritual aspirant; one who is striving on the spiritual path for self-realization and enlightenment by practising some form of sadhana

Sadhana – spiritual practice done regularly for attainment of experience and realization of the self, true reality and cosmic consciousness

Sahasrara chakra – thousand-petalled lotus at the top of the head, associated with the pituitary gland

Samadhi – final stage of meditation, state of oneness, unity with the object of meditation

Samana vayu – pranic air current of the middle region of the body, facilitates assimilation

Samskara – mental impressions stored in the subtle body and in the brain as archetypes

Sapta dhatu – the seven body minerals: bone, fat, flesh, blood, skin, marrow and semen/ova

Saptami – seventh day of the moon's waxing and waning

Saraswati nadi – to the right of sushumna running up to the tongue

Saraswati – subterranean holy river in India which converges with Ganga and Yamuna at Prayag, U.P.; associated with sushumna nadi in the body

Sattwa – third quality of nature and mind which is illumined, steady, pure and unwavering

Saumya nadi – travels to the tips of the toes

Shakti – vital energy force

Shankini nadi – on the left side running between saraswati and gandhari nadis

Shanmukhi mudra – particular mudra of closing the seven facial orifices with the fingers

Shasthami – sixth day of the moon, occurring twice a month

221

Shastra – an authoritative treatise on any subject, particularly science and religion

Shiva – state of pure consciousness, individual and cosmic

Shiva Swarodaya – Sanskrit text on the science of swara yoga

Shubha – auspicious

Shura nadi – from manipura to ajna chakras

Siddha – an adept, perfected one

Siddhi – perfection, activated pranic and psychic capacity

So-Ham – psychic sound of the breath; mantra for japa; So represents cosmic consciousness, Ham represents individual awareness and existence

Sthula sharira – gross physical body

Sukshma sharira – subtle or astral body

Surya nadi – sun or pingala nadi

Sushumna nadi – main central nadi in the spinal cord for channelling kundalini shakti

Sushupti – unconscious realm and state of mind, deep sleep

Swadhisthana chakra – second chakra up from mooladhara in the sacral plexus

Swapna – subconscious realm and state of mind, dream

Swara – the flow of air in one or two nostrils, also means sound or tone

Swarodaya – the beginning or rising time of the swara

Tamas – the first quality of nature, inertia

Tanmatra – subtle or primary essence, of gandha (smell), rasa (taste), roopa (form or sight), sparsha (feel or touch), shabda (speech or sound) from which the grosser elements or qualities are produced

Tantra – the oldest science and philosophy of man; the process of liberation and expansion of mind, energy and consciousness

Tattwa – element, true or real state

Tejas – fire or lustre, brilliance

Tejas tattwa – fire element, agni tattwa

Tithi – date, day of the moon's phase

Trataka – technique of steadily gazing at an object such as a candle flame, mandala or yantra

Trayodashi – thirteenth day of the moon's phases

Tritiya – third day of the moon's waxing and waning

Ucchatana – a kind of charm or magic incantation causing a person to leave his business in disgust

Udana – pranic air current in the throat and face

Upanishads – books of the Vedas, traditionally 108, which belong to the shruti or the revealed knowledge of guru to disciple; realizations of the rishis and sages concerning reality and the identity of individual consciousness

Upa prana – subsidiary prana functions

Upasana – concentration, dharana

Vajra nadi – first nadi inside sushumna representing rajas

Vama swara – left nostril activities when the flow of air passes through the left nostril

Varuni nadi – controls urination; located between kuhu and yashaswini nadis in the sacral plexus

Vashikaran – the art of fascinating, attracting, alluring, subduing or subjugating

Vayu – pranic air current

Vayu tattwa – air element

Vedas – most ancient books of man explaining every aspect of life from supreme reality to worldly affairs

Vidya – form of knowledge

Vijnanamaya kosha – sheath made of intuition or higher knowledge

Vilamabanadi – also known as the navel wheel, situated at manipura chakra

Virat – cosmic prana or cosmic body

Vishnu – one of the holy trinity, cosmic preserver; also said to reside in manipura chakra; vital capacity of manipura to stimulate and store prana so that health and stamina are maintained

Vishuddhi chakra – psychic and pranic energy centre in the cervical plexus

Vishwodari nadi – between kuhu and hastijihva nadis in the lower part of the body

Vyana – pranic air current pervading the whole body

Yamuna – famous holy river in India, yellow in colour; associated with pingala nadi in the body; Yamuna emerges in the

Himalayan mountains at Yamunotri and converges with Ganga and Saraswati in Uttar Pradesh, in a place known as Triveni; in some places Yamuna completely dries up in summer, just as prana also leaves the body

Yantra – precisely calculated geometrical symbol representing specific forces of shakti and consciousness, for example, Sri Yantra represents the creation and existence of the universe; a tool of tantra used to liberate energy and consciousness from mind and body

Yashaswini nadi – in front of pingala running from the right hand to the left leg

Yoga – state of union between two opposite poles; process of uniting the two opposite forces in the body in order to liberate the consciousness from the gross mind

Yoga danda – specially designed stick used by yogis which they rest in the armpit to change the flow of the swara

Yoni mudra – also known as shanmukhi mudra, closing the seven gates of perception in the head; also a hand mudra with the fingers forming the shape of the yoni or womb

Bibliography

Chapter 2

[1] 'Electronic evidence of auras/chakras in UCLA study', *Brain/Mind Bulletin*, March 20, 1987, 3(11).

[2] ibid.

Chapter 3

[1] Saxton, H., *The Fields of Life – Our Links with the Universe*, Ballantine Books, New York, 1972.

[2] Gauquelin, M., *The Cosmic Clocks*, Paladin, 1973.

[3] Ravitz, L.J., *Annals of the New York Academy of Sciences*, 98(4):114–20, 1962.

Motoyama, H., 'The mechanisms through which paranormal phenomena take place', *Religion and Parapsychology*, 1975, 2.

[4] Playfair, G.L. & Hill, S., *The Cycles of Heaven*, 2nd edn, Pan Books Ltd., 1979.

op. cit., Gauquelin.

[5] Kruegar, A. & Smith, R., 'The physiological significance of positive and negative ionization in the atmosphere', *Man's Dependence on the Earthly Atmosphere*, Macmillan, New York, 1962.

[6] op. cit., Playfair & Hill.

[7] Diamond, M.C., *Psychology Today*, June 1980.

[8] op. cit., Playfair & Hill.

Chapter 4

1. Riga, I.N., 'The neuro-reflex syndrome of unilateral nasal obstruction', *Revue D'Oto-Neuro- Opthalmologie*, 1957, 29(6).

2. ibid.

3. ibid.

4. Engen, T., 'Why the aroma lingers on', *Psychology Today*, May 1981.

5. Hopson, J., 'Smell, the provocative sense frontier', *Psychology Today*, May 1981. 'Menstrual rhythms synchronized among close companions, room-mates', *Brain/Mind Bulletin*, April 20, 1981, 6(8).

6. Bhole, M.V. & Karambelkar, P.V., 'Significance of nostrils in breathing', *Yoga Mimamsa*, 1968, X(4):1–12.

7. op. cit., Playfair & Hill.

Chapter 5

1. Nostrand, V., *The Philosophical Impact of Contemporary Physics*, Princeton, N.J.

Chapter 10

1. Motoyama, H., 'An electrophysiological study of prana (Ki)', *IARP Journal* 4(1):1–27, 1978.

2. Ornstein, R., *The Nature of Human Consciousness: A book of readings*, W.H. Freeman & Co., San Francisco, 1973.

3. Kinsbourne, M., Neurologist, 'Sad hemisphere, happy hemisphere', *Psychology Today*, May 1981.

4. 'Emotional quality of speech attributed to right brain', *Brain/Mind Bulletin*, May 7, 1979, 4(12).

'Personality disorders may reflect over-reliance on left or right brain', *Brain/Mind Bulletin*, Jan. 7, 1980, 5(4).

5. 'Sex differences in perception due to inherent biases', *Brain/Mind Bulletin*, Jan. 16, 1978, 3(5).

'Finches brains sexually altered', *Brain/Mind Bulletin*, Feb. 18, 1980, 5(7).

'Sex differences seen in brain asymmetries', *Brain/Mind Bulletin*, June 2, 1980, 5(14).

Chapter 12

[1] Motoyama, H., *Theories on the Chakras – bridges to higher consciousness*, Theosophical Publishing House, 1981.

Chapter 13

[1] Friedman, H., Becker, R. & Bachman, C., 'Geomagnetic parameters and psychiatric hospital admissions', *Nature*, CC 1963, 629.

Raman, B.V., *Lectures on Astrology*, University of Rajasthan Press, Jaipur, 1967.

'Statistical study finds tie between planets, personality', *Brain/Mind Bulletin*, Feb. 4, 1980, 5(6).

Chapter 17

[1] Chase, M.H., 'Every ninety minutes a brain storm', *Psychology Today*, Nov. 1979.

'Rhythm found for cognitive styles', *Brain/Mind Bulletin*, July 16, 1979, 4(17).

Goleman, D., Davidson, R.J., *Consciousness: Brain, States of Awareness and Mysticism*, Harper & Row Publishers, 1979.

[2] ibid., Goleman.

Chapter 18

[1] Luce, G.G., *Body Time*, Paladin, 1973.

Chapter 19

[1] Sing, H.G., 'Swara Vigyan and behaviour patterns', *Vedic Path*, March 1981.

[2] ibid.

Notes

— Notes —